A Guide to Hypertrophic Cardiomyopathy

A Guide to Hypertrophic Cardiomyopathy

For Patients, Their Families, and Interested Physicians

THIRD EDITION

Barry J. Maron, MD

Director, Hypertrophic Cardiomyopathy Center
Minneapolis Heart Institute Foundation
Minneapolis, MN, USA
Adjunct Professor of Medicine
Tufts University School of Medicine
Boston, MA, USA
Adjunct Professor of Medicine
Mayo Medical School
Rochester, MN, USA

Lisa Salberg

Chief Executive Officer and Founder
Hypertrophic Cardiomyopathy Association (HCMA)
Hibernia, NJ, USA

WILEY Blackwell

Registered Office
John Wiley & Sons, Ltd, The Atrium, Southern Gate, Chichester, West Sussex, PO19 8SQ, UK

Editorial Offices
9600 Garsington Road, Oxford, OX4 2DQ, UK
The Atrium, Southern Gate, Chichester, West Sussex, PO19 8SQ, UK
111 River Street, Hoboken, NJ 07030-5774, USA

For details of our global editorial offices, for customer services and for information about
how to apply for permission to reuse the copyright material in this book please see our website
at www.wiley.com/wiley-blackwell

Library of Congress Cataloging-in-Publication Data

Maron, Barry J. (Barry Joel), 1941- author.
  A guide to hypertrophic cardiomyopathy : for patients, their families, and interested physicians /
Barry J. Maron, Lisa Salberg. – Third edition.
      p. ; cm.
  Preceded by: Hypertrophic cardiomyopathy / by Barry J. Maron, Lisa Salberg. 2nd ed. 2006.
  Includes bibliographical references and index.
    ISBN 978-0-470-67504-5 (pbk. : alk. paper) – ISBN 978-1-118-72549-8 – ISBN 978-1-118-72551-1 –
ISBN 978-1-118-72552-8 (epdf) – ISBN 978-1-118-72553-5 (epub)
    I. Salberg, Lisa, author.   II. Maron, Barry J. (Barry Joel), 1941- Hypertrophic cardiomyopathy.
Preceded by (work):   III. Title.
  [DNLM: 1. Cardiomyopathy, Hypertrophic–Popular Works.   2. Patient Education as
Topic–Popular Works.   WG 280]
  RC685.H9
  616.1'24–dc23
                                                                                          2013026489

Cover image: Cover image courtesy of the authors.
Cover design by Andrew Magee Design Ltd.

Set in 9.5/13pt Meridien by SPi Publisher Services, Pondicherry, India

1   2014

Contents

- Obstructive sleep apnea and HCM, 78

- Gene therapy and stem cells, 78

- Automated external defibrillators (AEDs), 79

- HCM as a chronic disease: Is a cure available?, 80

- Are you newly diagnosed?, 82

- Adapting psychologically to HCM, 84

- Family screening, 87

- What about having children? Pregnancy and delivery, 89

- Routine medical care, 91

- Community screening for HCM, 96

- Community outreach, 97

- Driving, 98

- Traveling, 99

- Military service, 100

- Social security benefits, 101

- Family and Medical Leave Act, 103

- Health insurance, 103

- Life insurance, 105

- Students, 105

- HCM Centers, 106

- Support and advocacy groups (HCMA), 107

- What research is being conducted?, 110

- The 36 most frequently asked questions about HCM that are addressed to the HCMA by patients, caregivers, and family members, 112

Acknowledgments and Dedications

I would like to acknowledge the constant, unwavering, and good-natured support that made this book (and the many HCM papers) possible over 40 years from my wife, Donna, as well as our 2 sons, Dr. Martin Maron and Dr. Bradley Maron, both cardiologists in Boston. I also wish to recognize our 2 grandchildren, Alexis (age 9) and Jack (age 8), both brilliant and currently preparing applications to medical school and the MCAT examination.

Barry J. Maron, MD
Director, Hypertrophic Cardiomyopathy Center
Minneapolis Heart Institute Foundation
Minneapolis, MN, USA
Adjunct Professor of Medicine
Tufts University School of Medicine
Boston, MA, USA
Adjunct Professor of Medicine
Mayo Medical School
Rochester, MN, USA

*****

To those in my family lost to HCM – Dad, Lori, Tom, Alice, Grandpa Larry, Great Grandmother Mary, and others. To those who are living with clinical HCM – Becca, Stacey, John, and Patty. To those who carry the gene for HCM and wonder if it will someday impact them. To my larger HCMA family it is my sincere wish that this book aids in global understanding that one day leads to a cure so other families do not suffer as ours has.

Thank you to Kelly DeRosa, Carolyn Willis and the Board of Directors (past and present) for their dedication to the HCMA and our mission.

To Adam and Becca I love you both to the moon and back... Always.

Lisa Salberg
Founder and CEO
Hypertrophic Cardiomyopathy Association

Foreword

More than a half century ago, when I was a young cardiologist at the National Institutes of Health (NIH), my colleagues and I encountered two young men with obstruction to the outflow of blood from the heart's main pumping chamber, the left ventricle. The condition was quite mysterious since the cause of the obstruction was not clear and the available medical literature was unhelpful. With the passage of time, our group at the NIH and other cardiologists and cardiovascular surgeons around the world recognized an increasing number of such patients and learned that this condition, now called hypertrophic cardiomyopathy (HCM), could present in a wide variety of ways. However, it was thought at first that obstruction was a *sine qua non* of HCM and that the prognosis was guarded.

As a result of extensive and carefully conducted research by many talented scientists and clinicians, the veil surrounding this condition has been lifted, and we now know that rather than a medical curiosity, HCM is, in fact, the most common genetic cardiac disease. It occurs in approximately 1 of every 500 persons, more than a half million patients in the United States alone. The abnormal genes responsible in the majority of patients with HCM have been discovered and can be tested for. Screening and diagnosis can be accomplished readily with an ultrasound examination. Perhaps most important, it has been established that most patients can lead normal or near normal lives. Management can be "tailored" to individual patients; many require nothing more than lifestyle modification and careful follow up examinations. In other patients symptoms can be managed with commonly used drugs, such as the familiar beta blockers. Serious disturbances of cardiac rhythm can now be aborted with an implanted defibrillator. An operation, surgical myomectomy, pioneered at the NIH more than fifty years ago, is reserved for patients with severe symptomatic obstruction and has improved steadily over the years. The risk of the procedure is now very low when it is carried out in experienced institutions. Alcohol septal ablation, carried out in the cardiac catheterization laboratory, is an alternative treatment of obstruction. Both procedures must be performed by experts.

This exceptionally well written "short book" on HCM describes the nature of the disease, the implications of genetic transmission, as well as the methods of screening, diagnosis and estimating prognosis. All forms of treatment, their indications and risks are discussed. Importantly, this book provides useful recommendations on lifestyle, sports and pregnancy.

The authors bring their extensive experience to this book. Dr. Maron has devoted his professional life to the study of and research into HCM and is considered a world authority on this condition. He shares his immense knowledge with the reader. Ms. Salberg, a patient with HCM, who is the founder and President of the HCM Association, provides the critically important perspectives of patients and their families. This lucid and understandable book will be of enormous value to patients with HCM, their families and caregivers, including physicians. Dr. Maron and Ms. Salberg deserve profound thanks for devoting their effort and talent to this important project.

Eugene Braunwald, M.D.
Brigham and Women's Hospital
Harvard Medical School
Boston, Massachusetts

Introduction: Tips for using this book

If you are reading this book, you probably fall into three potential groups: (1) you have HCM, (2) a friend or relative has HCM, or (3) you are a healthcare provider. An effort has been made here to inform each of these groups about HCM in language that is only as scientific as necessary yet at the same time comprehensive, up to date, and complete. Each section of the book is similar with a narrative explanation of the topic and a boxed summary message, where appropriate, at the end of each section. This is intended as a "take home message" to patients and families.

As with the prior two editions, this updated version of the book is a collaboration between Dr. Barry J. Maron, an authority with a unique interest in HCM over almost 40 years, and Lisa Salberg, a patient with HCM and the Founder and CEO of the Hypertrophic Cardiomyopathy Association (HCMA) – a patient advocacy organization devoted to this disease. Therefore, this book blends scientific data with a first person perspective of this disease.

HCM patients (and their cardiologists) found prior editions of the book helpful and enlightening by offering clarity and guidance. This is particularly important for a complex disease such as HCM, which has attracted so much misunderstanding and uncertainty over the last five decades.

Disease Principles for HCM:

- Heterogeneity
- Unpredictability
- Often without absolute certainty

What is hypertrophic cardiomyopathy (HCM)

Cardiomyopathy is a general term describing any condition in which the heart muscle is structurally and functionally abnormal (the heart itself is, of course, a specialized type of muscle). While there are many types of cardiomyopathy (e.g., dilated, restrictive, and right ventricular), many of which are genetic and familial, we are concerned here with only *hypertrophic cardiomyopathy (HCM)*.

HCM is a genetic disease affecting the heart muscle. The most consistent feature of HCM is excessive thickening (*hypertrophy*) of that portion of the heart known as the left ventricle. In quantitative terms, hypertrophy is usually defined as a wall thickness of 15 mm or more when measured by ultrasound (echocardiogram) or cardiac magnetic resonance imaging (MRI), but any wall thickness (including normal) is consistent with the presence of a gene causing HCM. The consequences of HCM to patients are related, in part or solely, to the abnormally thickened left ventricular heart muscle, which in turn is a consequence of the basic genetic defect. Hypertrophy may be widespread throughout the left ventricle, but may also be more limited in distribution, involving only very small portions of the wall; there is no single pattern of muscle thickening which is "typical" for HCM. The region of the left ventricle which is usually the site of the most prominent thickening is the *ventricular septum*, that is, that portion of muscle which separates the left and right ventricular cavities. These patterns of hypertrophy do not represent separate disease states, but are all part of the HCM spectrum.

The heart (specifically the left ventricle) may also thicken in other individuals who do not have HCM, either as a result of high blood pressure, obstructive heart valve disease, or even occasionally with prolonged and intense athletic training in certain sports. The type of hypertrophy of the left ventricle associated with high blood pressure is often referred to as *secondary* (i.e., a consequence of the increased blood pressure). In HCM,

A Guide to Hypertrophic Cardiomyopathy: For Patients, Their Families, and Interested Physicians, Third Edition. Barry J. Maron and Lisa Salberg.
© 2014 John Wiley & Sons, Ltd. Published 2014 by John Wiley & Sons, Ltd.

(a)

(b)

(c)

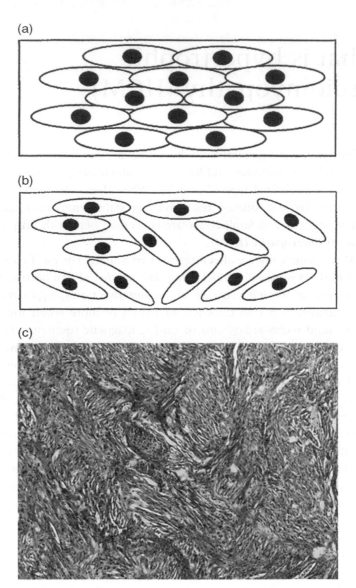

Figure 1 The cell structure and architecture of the HCM heart. Diagrams contrast (a) the regular and parallel alignment of cardiac muscle cells characteristic of the normal heart with (b) the irregular, disorganized alignment of cells ("myocardial disarray") found in some areas of the HCM heart. At the bottom is a micrograph from an HCM heart (i.e., histologic section) showing the disorganized and chaotic arrangement of cardiac muscle cells (myocytes) (c).

however, the muscular thickening of the heart wall is *primary* – that is, due to a genetic defect and not a reaction to other factors.

In addition, when the heart muscle of HCM is viewed under a light microscope, it usually shows several particular abnormalities, the most prominent of which is **myocardial cell (myocyte) disarray or disorganization**, in which the normal parallel alignment of heart muscle cells has been lost and many of the muscle cells are arranged in characteristically chaotic and disorganized patterns (Figure 1). It is likely that this cell disarray interferes with normal electrical transmission of impulses and predisposes some patients to irregularities of heart rhythm (and sudden death), as well as altering heart contraction. In addition, there are often collagen scars (i.e., areas of fibrosis of various size and extent within the left ventricular wall), which probably result from inadequate blood supply to the heart muscle.

- HCM is a common genetic cardiac disease causing the heart wall to thicken without enlarging the cavities.
- HCM is diverse in its presentation.
- Some people with thick hearts may not have HCM and instead the thickness may result from high blood pressure, valve disease, or prolonged athletic training.

Historical perspective and names

The first modern description of HCM was in 1958 by a British pathologist, Dr. Donald Teare, who likened the disease to a tumor of the heart. However, there is some evidence that HCM was initially recognized in the mid-1850s by German and French investigators. Nevertheless, over these many years, the condition has been known by a vast number of names. Indeed, this issue of nomenclature *is* often confusing to patients and even some physicians.

Remarkably, HCM has been given over 75 separate names by individual clinicians and scientists over the last 50 years (Figure 2). Literally, no other disease can make that claim. Why has this occurred? The principal reason for the proliferation of names undoubtedly has been the clinical heterogeneity and diversity with which HCM is expressed, a major point in ultimately understanding this disease. Also, since very

Asymmetrical hypertrophic cardiomyopathy
Asymmetrical hypertrophy of the heart
Asymmetrical septal hypertrophy
Brock's disease
Diffuse muscular subaortic stenosis
Diffuse subvalvular aortic stenosis
Dynamic hypertrophic subaortic stenosis
Dynamic muscular subaortic stenosis
Familial hypertrophic subaortic stenosis
Familial hypertrophic cardiomyopathy
Familial muscular subaortic stenosis
Familial myocardial disease
Functional aortic stenosis
Functional hypertrophic subaortic stenosis
Functional obstructive cardiomyopathy
Functional obstruction of the left ventricle
Functional obstructive subvalvular aortic stenosis
Functional subaortic stenosis
Hereditary cardiovascular dysplasia
HYPERTROPHIC CARDIOMYOPATHY (HCM)
Hypertrophic constrictive cardiomyopathy
Hypertrophic hyperkinetic cardiomyopathy
Hypertrophic infundibular aortic stenosis
Hypertrophic nonobstructive cardiomyopathy
Hypertrophic obstructive cardiomyopathy (HOCM)
Hypertrophic stenosing cardiomyopathy
Hypertrophic subaortic stenosis
Idiopathic hypertrophic cardiomyopathy
Idiopathic hypertrophic obstructive cardiomyopathy
Idiopathic hypertrophic subaortic stenosis (IHSS)

Idiopathic hypertrophic subvalvular stenosis
Idiopathic muscular hypertrophic subaortic stenosis
Idiopathic muscular stenosis of the left ventricle
Idiopathic myocardial hypertrophy
Idiopathic stenosis of the flushing chamber of LV
Idiopathic ventricular septal hypertrophy
Irregular hypertrophic cardiomyopathy
Left ventricular muscular stenosis
Low subvalvular aortic stenosis
Muscular aortic stenosis
Muscular hypertrophic stenosis of LV
Muscular stenosis of the left ventricle
Muscular subaortic stenosis
Muscular subvalvular aortic stenosis
Non-dilated cardiomyopathy
Nonobstructive hypertrophic cardiomyopathy
Obstructive cardiomyopathy
Obstructive hypertrophic aortic stenosis
Obstructive hypertrophic cardiomyopathy
Obstructive hypertrophic myocardiopathy
Obstructive myocardiopathy
Pseudoaortic stenosis
Stenosing hypertrophy of the left ventricle
Stenosis of the ejection chamber of LV
Subaortic hypertrophic stenosis
Subaortic idiopathic stenosis
Subaortic muscular stenosis
Subvalvular aortic stenosis of the muscular type
Teare's disease

Figure 2 Hypertrophic cardiomyopathy has acquired many names (about 75) in four decades, which primarily reflects the diversity with which the disease is expressed. Hypertrophic cardiomyopathy (HCM) is the preferred name at this time.

few cardiologists have treated large numbers of patients with HCM, they often came to regard the overall disease based solely on their personal (and sometimes limited) experiences.

Many of the alternate names for HCM emphasize obstruction to left ventricular outflow, which is a highly visible feature of the disease. Obstruction is probably present under resting conditions in just 25% of all patients; however, about 70% of all HCM patients have the capacity to generate obstruction, either at rest or (if not present at rest) when provoked by physiologic exercise. Therefore, names for this disease in the past have included idiopathic hypertrophic subaortic (*stenosis*) (IHSS), which was the first popular term used in the United States ("stenosis" means obstruction). The same can be said for hypertrophic obstructive cardiomyopathy (HOCM), which is still widely used in the United Kingdom. Indeed, you may well hear your disease referred to by more than the currently accepted designation – *HCM*.

Indeed, virtually all HCM experts and other cardiovascular specialists now regard *HCM* as the single best name for the broad disease spectrum. The term combines *hypertrophy* (which is the diagnostic marker in most patients) with the fact that this disease is a *cardiomyopathy* (or heart muscle disorder), and furthermore excludes specific reference to obstruction (which is *not* present in all patients). Therefore, the terms "HCM *with* obstruction" or "HCM *without* obstruction" are preferred.

HCM is a *genetic* disease based on the recognition 20 years ago that it is caused by mutations in genes coding proteins in the heart muscle. It is also a *familial* disease because it is transmitted to every generation as a dominant trait (i.e., about 50% of each generation are at risk). HCM is usually *inherited*, but there is also a phenomenon of *de novo* mutation when the disease (and mutation) appears for the first time in a family. It is probably not proper to consider HCM a *congenital* heart disease since it is only the disease-causing mutation which is always present from birth.

- HCM has had many names in the past.
- Hypertrophic cardiomyopathy or "HCM" is the preferred terminology.

How common is HCM?

HCM has had a misleading reputation as a rare disease. It is global in distribution, reported from all continents and more than 50 countries. However, a number of recent population studies from the United States and elsewhere in the world show that HCM is a much more common disease than previously regarded. It is now estimated that at least about 1 in 500 individuals within the general population are affected by this disease, equivalent to about 750,000 Americans (Figure 3). HCM is truly a global disease and these prevalence figures come from populations as diverse as the United States, Japan, Africa, and China. These figures relate to adults in whom the disease is recognized by echocardiography (i.e., by visualizing the thickening of the left ventricular wall). However, many other children and adults could carry a mutant gene for HCM and not be easily detectable by echocardiography or not come to clinical recognition for a variety of reasons (including absence of a heart murmur and obstruction), and therefore may be completely unaware of their diagnosis. Indeed, the 1 in 500 prevalence figure is likely to be an *underestimate* given the large number of genetically affected individuals in HCM families with little or no overt clinical evidence of the disease.

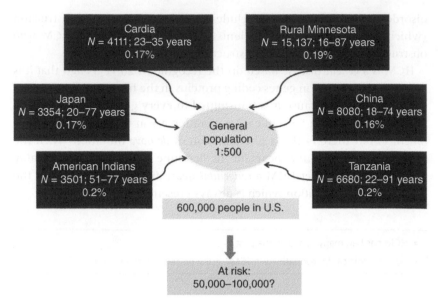

Figure 3 The reported prevalence of 1:500 for HCM is based on actual population data from different parts of the world.

Indeed, the currently recognized HCM patient population has been likened to the "tip of the iceberg," with most affected patients undiagnosed and "below the surface" (Figure 4). This helps explain why HCM seems so uncommon in cardiology practice, that is, why cardiologists so often tell HCM patients that they only occasionally see this condition.

The large number of names used to describe HCM may be one factor responsible for the perceived low visibility of HCM in the public sector relative to other less common diseases. In fact, HCM is much more common, and has more impact on the public health, than more visible noncardiac conditions such as cystic fibrosis, multiple sclerosis, muscular dystrophy, and amyotrophic lateral sclerosis (ALS; Lou Gehrig disease), or cardiovascular diseases such as Marfan syndrome (Figure 5). These other conditions are truly rare, occurring in only 1:10,000 or less of the general population while HCM is the most common genetic heart disease and most frequent cause of sudden death in the young – occurring in 1:500 people (Figure 5).

HCM occurs throughout the world (Figure 6), with most of the scientific interest and reports from North America (United States and Canada), the Far East (Japan, China, Australia), and Europe (United Kingdom, Italy, France, Germany, Switzerland), although there is increasing attention to HCM in Brazil, Argentina, Chile, Israel, and New Zealand. HCM appears to be remarkably similar with regard to its clinical presentation, heart

HCM: The tip of the iceberg

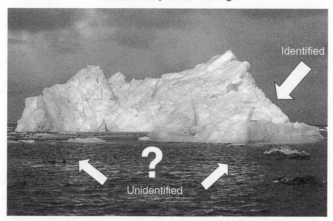

Figure 4 The HCM patients who are currently recognized clinically represent the "tip of the iceberg" – that is, a minority of the overall HCM population. Therefore, most HCM patients remain undiagnosed.

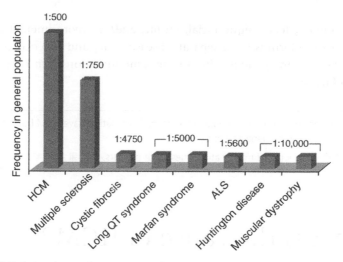

Figure 5 Relative disease frequencies in the general population, including for HCM. Other genetic cardiac or noncardiac diseases have assumed much greater public visibility, but among all these diseases, HCM is distinctly more common.
ALS = amyotrophic lateral sclerosis.

structure, clinical course, and prognosis in patients from these diverse areas of the world. One relatively minor exception is the apical form of HCM with wall thickening localized to the tip [apex] of the left ventricle, always without obstruction, which seems to be more common in Japan – a distinction

HCM is a global disease

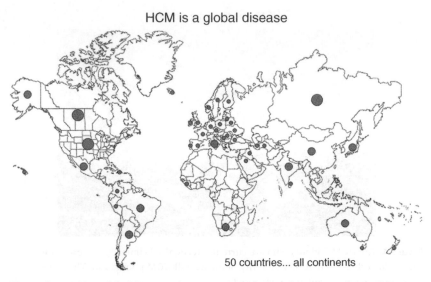

50 countries... all continents

Figure 6 HCM is a global disease. The expression of HCM throughout the world is largely the same.

which could reflect unique racial, ethnic, and/or environmental factors. This structural form is not a separate disease entity and also occurs in 3% of US (non-Asian) patients, due to the same mutations that cause other forms of HCM.

- HCM is common; 1 in 500 people in the general population have HCM but many more may carry the gene and not be aware.
- HCM affects people of many nationalities, both genders, and all ages.

What is the cause of HCM?

As emphasized earlier, HCM is a genetically transmitted and usually familial condition. The pattern of inheritance of HCM is known as *autosomal-dominant*, which means that the disease (and the mutant gene) occurs in about 50% of the relatives in each consecutive generation (Figure 7). Therefore, the likelihood of an affected parent transmitting the abnormal gene to their child is statistically about one in two. However, autosomal-dominant inheritance does not necessarily mean that in each

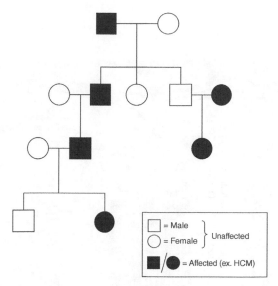

Figure 7 Family tree. Shown here are four generations of a family affected by HCM. There is a typical autosomal-dominant inheritance in which the condition is transmitted from one generation to another. In each generation, every offspring of an affected person has statistically a 50% chance of inheriting the gene or disease.

family if there are four offspring, two must be affected – only that this is the statistical probability. In reality, it could be zero of four or even four of four offspring who will carry the mutant gene. In addition, some individuals with this disease appear to be "sporadic" cases – that is, there are no other relatives in the family known to have evidence of HCM. There is always the possibility of a *de novo* (new) mutation – that is, the first member of the family with the mutant gene and expressed disease.

Genetic "skipping" of a generation is rare but can appear to occur when an individual who is a gene carrier does not have evidence of HCM on the echocardiogram. In such a circumstance, the defective gene does not actually "skip" a generation – but in reality the HCM gene in that individual simply does not express itself fully so that evidence of the disease cannot be visualized with the echocardiogram or MRI (known as *incomplete penetrance*).

A multitude of more than 1500 mutations in 11 genes, necessary for the development and contraction of heart muscle cells (in units called **sarcomeres**), have been mapped and isolated from members of families with HCM. The 11 genes currently known to cause HCM are (1) beta-myosin heavy chain; (2) myosin-binding protein C; (3) troponin-T; (4) troponin-I; (5) troponin-C; (6) alpha-tropomyosin; (7) and (8) essential and regulatory myosin light chains; (9) actin; (10) actin-2; and (11) myozenin-2 (Figure 8).

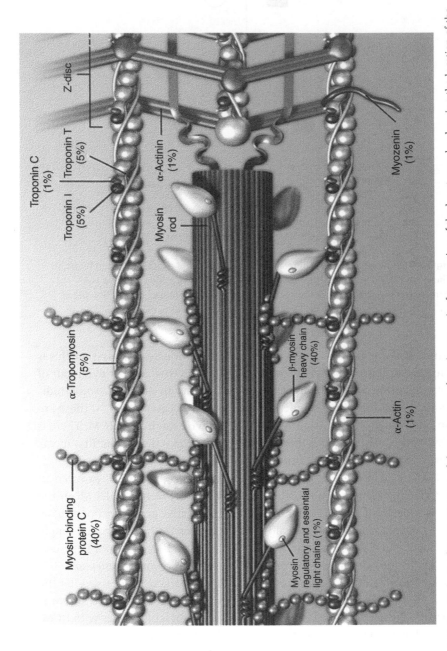

Figure 8 Genetic basis of HCM. Diagram of the sarcomere, the primary unit of contraction of the heart muscle, showing the location of the genes known to be responsible for HCM, with their frequency noted in parentheses.

Most commonly, HCM is caused by the first two genes on this list while the other nine genes each account for only a small fraction of the patients. Indeed, this is one of the reasons HCM is widely regarded as a diverse and heterogeneous disease. Additional genes and mutations responsible for HCM will be identified in the future since the known mutant genes account for only about 50% of the overall patient population. Not finding a gene mutation does not mean that the test subject does not have HCM, only that they do not carry one of the known mutations.

A **mutation** is a defect in the deoxyribonucleic acid (DNA) code, the protein structure of the gene. These DNA abnormalities may take many forms, but some can be likened to a "spelling error" in the genetic code of DNA, such as displacement in the order or sequence of just one of the many amino acids (the individual "building blocks" of the gene protein). Indeed, it is perhaps surprising that such seemingly minor-appearing abnormalities in the gene sequence can make such a profound difference in the structure of the heart, as occurs in HCM.

Patients often ask about the cause of their mutation, particularly if the gene abnormality has apparently appeared for the first time in a family. This consideration usually arises when a newly diagnosed child has both parents with normal echocardiograms and no evidence of HCM. Keep in mind that the genetic predisposition to HCM does not always trace back many generations in the same family, but may occur spontaneously for the first time in a member of the most recent generation. At present, the environmental factors that trigger HCM mutations are unknown.

The discovery of the gene defects responsible for HCM (more than 20 years ago) is a major step toward understanding the basic cause of HCM. In addition, laboratory DNA diagnosis from a blood test is now available for the first time commercially from four companies (Table 1). This availability can prove useful in identifying risk for HCM in young family members, in patients with systemic hypertension, or in clinical situations where the HCM diagnosis is ambiguous – such as athletes in whom it may be difficult to distinguish HCM from the physiologic effects of chronic exercise and training on the heart (i.e., "athlete's heart").

Most importantly, genetic testing has been utilized selectively by families with a known HCM mutation to determine if their children or other relatives without hypertrophy carry the same genetic marker (Figure 9). This knowledge will allow for careful follow-up for those with the mutation or, alternatively, freedom from the need for annual cardiac evaluation in those relatives without the mutation. Knowledge of a "mutation" may be highly emotional, debilitating, and, in some ways, even worse than an

Table 1 Commercial genetic testing services in the United States for HCM.

Company	Began HCM testing (year)	Website	Telephone	Number of HCM genes in panel	Turnaround time (weeks)	Number of probability categories	Genetic consultation available*	Variant reclassification	Cost (proband testing)	Cost (other family members)	Number of other genetic diseases tested
GeneDx (Gaithersburg, MD)	2008	www.genedx.com	301-519-2100	18	8	5	+	+	$3375*	$350	350
Transgenomic-FAMILION (New Haven, CT)	2008	www.familion.com	877-274-9432	12	4–6	3	+	+	$5400	$900	10
Correlaen Diagnostics (Waltham, MA)	2007	www.correlagen.com	866-647-0735	16	6–8	7	+	+	$3975	$250	40
Partners (Cambridge, MA)	2003	www.pcpgm.partners.org	617-768-8500	18	5	5	+	+	$3200	$400	100

*Insurance program limits patient cost to $100, where this policy is permissible under local and state laws.

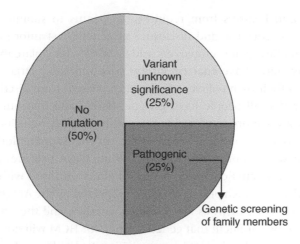

Figure 9 What can be expected from genetic testing? About 65–75% of the time, the result is not "actionable," meaning that the data in the report cannot be used to screen family members reliably – that is, either no mutation is found or the mutation that is identified is not known to actually cause HCM ("variant of unknown significance"). Only when the mutation is judged "pathogenic" (responsible for HCM in that family) can the genetic screening of family members proceed. The latter possibility can, however, be very powerful by definitively excluding relatives from the risk of developing HCM.

actual diagnosis for a particular patient. Genetic counseling is highly recommended for family members undergoing molecular screening to prepare them for the results and help interpret the findings.

Ongoing and future investigations will focus on the identification of new genes that cause HCM and ultimately how these genetic abnormalities operate in formulating HCM. Some molecular biologists believe that knowledge of the basic genetic defect in HCM will ultimately unlock many of the secrets of this disease and permit more targeted and earlier therapeutic interventions. However, such a level of understanding has not yet materialized. Cardiologists will continue to advise and treat patients with the available practical, clinical strategies – most of which have proven to be powerful and effective.

In May 2008, the Genetic Information Non-Discrimination Act (GINA) was signed into law in the United States. The Act prohibits discrimination on the basis of genetic information with respect to health insurance and employment. GINA also prevents health insurers from denying coverage or adjusting premiums based on an individual's predisposition to a genetic condition, and prohibits employers from discriminating on the basis of predictive (prognostic) genetic information. Additionally, GINA restrains both employers and insurers from requiring applicants to submit to genetic tests, requires strict use and disclosure of genetic test information, and imposes penalties against employers and insurers who violate these provisions. Many states have enacted similar laws and some large employers have created their own policies to protect employees from discrimination.

It is clear that all people have genetic "flaws" and that our society is moving toward a more comfortable relationship with genetic information. While cases of discrimination are rare, the fear of discrimination has been a key factor suppressing genetic testing. While GINA provides protection for those with a genetic marker, it has no effect on those with clinically identified diseases. Such protection may be covered by the Americans with Disability Act. With GINA as law, patients, families, and their health-care providers can be confident that genetic testing for HCM will not have negative consequences for those who test positive. It should also be noted that GINA does *not* provide protection from discrimination in life insurance or long-term disability policies.

- HCM is a genetic condition.
- Genetic testing for HCM is widely available.
- GINA protects genetic information from being used against anyone in the areas of health insurance or employment.
- HCM may mimic other conditions with hypertrophy, and different treatment strategies and genetic testing can help resolve these.

Structure of the heart

The normal heart

First, it is useful to review the structure and function of the normal heart in order to understand the abnormalities that occur in HCM (Figure 10). A normal heart has four heart chambers (left and right ventricles as the lower chambers; left and right atria as the upper chambers) and four valves (mitral and tricuspid; aortic and pulmonic). The walls of the heart are composed of muscle cells (myocytes), as well as collagen and small veins and arteries (called venules and arterioles, respectively). The left ventricular

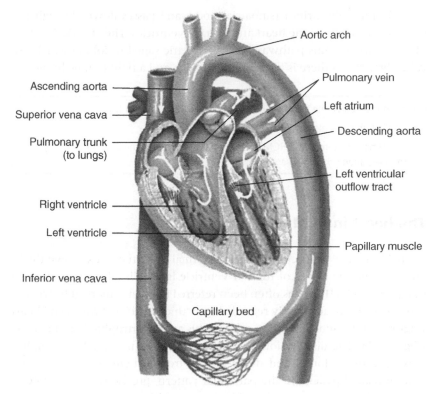

Aortic arch

Ascending aorta

Pulmonary vein

Left atrium

Superior vena cava

Descending aorta

Pulmonary trunk
(to lungs)

Left ventricular
outflow tract

Right ventricle

Left ventricle

Papillary muscle

Inferior vena cava

Capillary bed

Figure 10 Normal heart structure. It is helpful to be familiar with the structure and function of the normal heart in order to understand the abnormalities in HCM. This drawing shows a normal heart with heart chambers, valves, and the direction of blood flow. The walls of the heart are composed of specialized muscle known as myocardium. The arrows show the direction of blood flow through the heart. The right atrium receives blood from the body, transfers it to the right ventricle, which pumps it into the lungs to receive oxygen. This oxygenated blood returns to the heart from the lungs into the left atrium, to the left ventricle (through the mitral valve), which then pumps it into the systemic circulation through the aortic valve via the aorta.

wall is usually of similar thickness in all areas, and in normal adults measures 12 mm or less on the echocardiogram or MRI (in the relaxation phase of the cardiac cycle – i.e., diastole). The normal human heart weighs between 7 and 15 ounces (200–425 g) and is a little larger than the size of a fist. Size will vary based on gender, age, and body mass of the individual.

Systole is the contraction phase of the heart cycle and diastole is when the heart relaxes. The normal course of blood flow through the heart is shown in Figure 10. Every normal heartbeat results from an electrical signal which starts in the right atrium (sinoatrial node) and passes down through the conduction system of the heart and into the ventricles. The electrical system of the heart contains pathways for the electric signal to follow which are called branches – there is a left bundle branch and a right bundle branch.

- In normal hearts, the thickness of the left ventricle is 12 mm or less.
- In HCM, the wall measures 15–60 mm.
- Abnormal structure in the HCM heart may also include the mitral valve, papillary muscles, and/or the right ventricle.

The heart in HCM

In HCM, the left ventricular wall is abnormal by virtue of excessive thickening, while the cavity of the left ventricle is usually of normal or small size (Figure 11). HCM has often been referred to as an "enlarged heart" but is probably more accurately regarded as a "thickened" or "muscular" heart (Figure 12). Cardiologists may refer to this as "hypertrophied–nondilated" (Figure 13). The distribution of this muscle thickening (or hypertrophy) may take many forms and differ greatly from patient to patient (even among related patients). The particular pattern, precise site, or degree of hypertrophy may vary considerably among patients.

In addition, the absolute thickness of the wall may vary greatly among patients as well. HCM may reach thicknesses that far exceed those reported in any other cardiac disease – ranging up to six times the normal. The upper limit of normal wall thickness is 10–12 mm and, remarkably, some patients may show thickness as much as 40–60 mm. There can also be abnormal size and function of the mitral valve and location of papillary muscles. Most anatomic abnormalities of the heart are in the left ventricle, although many patients with HCM may have enlargement of the left atria, and rarely hypertrophy of the right ventricle.

Patients are often very focused on the exact "number" of their wall thickness, but actually in most patients this precise value is of limited significance clinically. One exception would be those with an extremely thick wall of 30 mm or more, which has been associated with increased risk for sudden death. On the other hand, many patients have only mildly increased thickness, which may be confined to only a small portion of the left ventricular wall.

Usually, hypertrophy in HCM is described as **asymmetric**, which means some parts of the wall are thicker than others. It is usually the ventricular septum which is the thickest, and portions of the left ventricular free wall

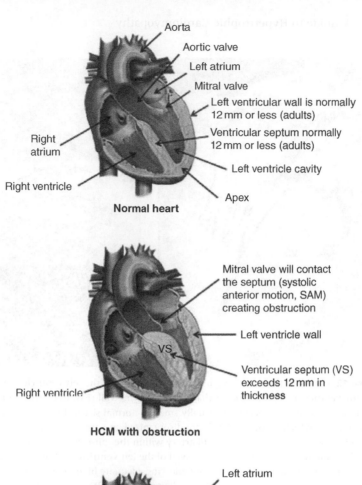

Normal heart

Aorta
Aortic valve
Left atrium
Mitral valve
Left ventricular wall is normally 12 mm or less (adults)
Ventricular septum normally 12 mm or less (adults)
Left ventricle cavity
Apex
Right ventricle
Right atrium

HCM with obstruction

Mitral valve will contact the septum (systolic anterior motion, SAM) creating obstruction
Left ventricle wall
VS
Ventricular septum (VS) exceeds 12 mm in thickness
Right ventricle

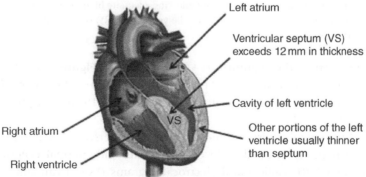

HCM without obstruction

Left atrium
Ventricular septum (VS) exceeds 12 mm in thickness
Cavity of left ventricle
VS
Other portions of the left ventricle usually thinner than septum
Right atrium
Right ventricle

Figure 11 Heart structure in HCM. Compared to normal (top), the HCM heart usually shows thickening of the ventricular septum which is greater than other areas of the left ventricular (LV) wall, whether or not there is obstruction (middle and bottom). However, the exact pattern of hypertrophy in HCM can be quite diverse and is not limited to that shown here. Obstruction occurs when the mitral valve comes forward and contacts the septum (arrow) – that is, systolic anterior motion of the mitral valve (SAM), as shown in the middle panel.

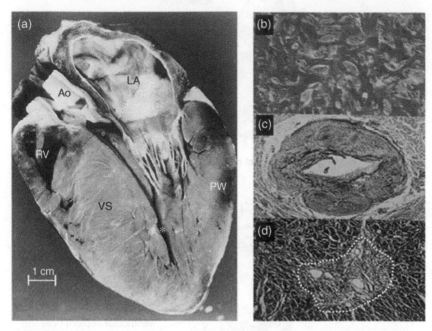

Figure 12 The HCM heart. (a) "Asymmetric" thickening of the left ventricle is evident with the ventricular septum thicker than the rest of the wall (FW, free wall). In HCM the cavity of the left ventricle (*) is usually small or normal sized. (b) Disorganized architecture in which myocardial cells are disorganized and arranged at perpendicular and oblique angles. (c) Abnormal small artery within the muscle with narrow aperture and thick wall. (d) Scar formation in the wall of the left ventricle that probably results because the narrowed artery in (b) is not allowing adequate blood flow to the heart muscle. Ao, aorta; LA, left atrium; MV, middle ventricular; RV, right ventricle; VS, ventricular septum.

(i.e., not part of the septum) are usually thinner (Figure 12). The term "concentric" only means that all portions of the wall are of the same thickness; this pattern of hypertrophy is uncommon in HCM, and present in only about 2% of patients.

HCM is a complex disease, and this point is underscored by the fact that a few genetically affected children and adults with normal echocardiograms (and MRI studies) and electrocardiograms (ECGs) can completely escape clinical recognition. Indeed, this is an example of *HCM without hypertrophy* (also known as "gene-positive–phenotype-negative"), which can be diagnosed only with genetic testing. However, based on available information, there does not seem to be significant risk associated with this expression of HCM, although many of these individuals may ultimately "convert" to a more typical appearance of HCM by developing a thick heart wall.

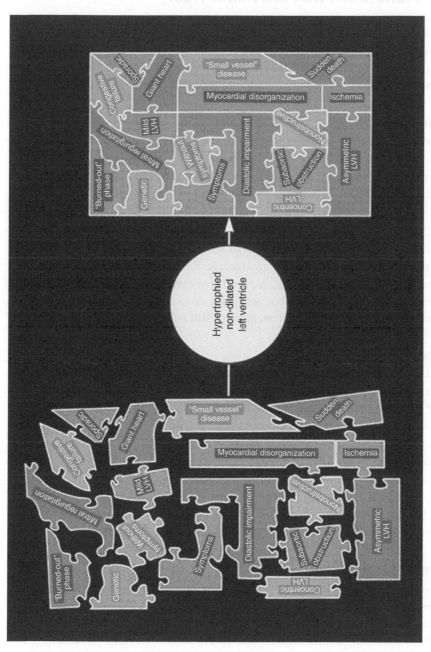

Figure 13 The clinical definition of HCM is based on the presence of left ventricular hypertrophy (LVH) without enlargement of either ventricular cavity in a patient who does not have another cardiac (or systemic) disease that itself could potentially produce the degree of hypertrophy evident in that patient. This is the basic criterion for diagnosis that brings together the diverse pieces of the jigsaw puzzle, which HCM often appears to be.

Heart conditions that can mimic HCM

In selected patients, it may become important for "real" HCM to be distinguished from a number of other cardiovascular conditions that can mimic the appearance of HCM. This may represent a complex clinical situation, probably most reliably resolved in a specialized HCM Center.

Athlete's heart

Occasionally systematic training in certain sports can thicken the left ventricle modestly, but sufficient to cause confusion with a HCM diagnosis. There are a number of noninvasive strategies that can resolve this issue, including a period of forced deconditioning (best assessed with repeat MRIs).

Left ventricular noncompaction

This designation means that portions of the heart (left ventricle) appear "spongy" and not compact as is characteristic of HCM. This appearance can represent a separate disease or occur in association with other cardiac diseases, including HCM. Because noncompaction is newly described, its natural history and treatment strategies are still being resolved.

Systemic hypertension

High blood pressure is a common problem in the general population. However, when hypertension is present in a patient suspected of having HCM, it can make the HCM diagnosis difficult. Nevertheless, when this dilemma arises, it is prudent to recommend family screening for HCM as a precaution.

Noonan disease

This is a separate disease entity which has distinctive facial characterization. A large percentage of these patients will have thickening of the left ventricle on echocardiogram which looks very much like HCM. The long-term clinical course of Noonan patients with hypertrophy is largely unknown.

LAMP2 (Danon disease)

This is a metabolic disorder that results in extreme hypertrophy of the left ventricle, often associated with a conduction abnormality known as Wolff–Parkinson–White. LAMP2 is a storage condition in which lysosome-degraded material accumulates in the heart. It is important to identify LAMP2 as this disease is much more severe than HCM with greatly impaired heart function – and survival beyond 25 years is unusual (for males). As LAMP2 is usually unresponsive to defibrillator therapy, heart transplantation is the sole effective treatment for LAMP2, and genetic testing is the only method of diagnosis.

Fabry disease

Fabry is another storage disease that can mimic HCM with left ventricular hypertrophy. Distinguishing Fabry from HCM is particularly important since treatment for Fabry is completely different and unique, involving (costly) enzyme replacement therapy. Fabry also can affect multiple organs other than the heart, particularly the kidney.

Pompe disease

Pompe is a rare inherited neuromuscular disorder that causes progressive muscle weakness in people of all ages, confusion between HCM and Pompe is reserved to the infantile presentation. The disease is named after Johannes C. Pompe, a Dutch physician who first described the disorder in 1932 in an infant patient. Pompe disease is caused by a defective gene that results in a deficiency of an enzyme, acid alpha-glucosidase (pronounced "AL-fa glue-CO-sih-days" and often abbreviated as **GAA**). The absence of this enzyme results in excessive buildup of a substance called glycogen, a form of sugar that is stored in a specialized compartment of muscle cells throughout the body. When this buildup occurs in the heart, there can be confusion with HCM.

Heart function in HCM

The thickened muscle of the left ventricle in HCM usually contracts well in the presence of small, or normal-sized, heart chambers – sometimes even better than normal – and rapidly ejects most of the blood from the heart (i.e., in systole). There are no particular adverse or beneficial implications to having a ventricle that contracts in this way. Only very few HCM patients develop depressed contraction associated with severe heart failure (as will be discussed later).

However, the heart muscle in HCM is often stiff and relaxes poorly when blood enters the ventricles passively during diastole (i.e., relaxation). It is believed that symptoms in HCM (such as shortness of breath with exercise) can be related, at least in part, to this impaired filling of the ventricles or obstruction. Therefore, the type of "heart failure" characteristic of HCM in which the heart actually contracts normally is very different from the much more common situation (due to coronary heart disease and heart attacks, or long-standing high blood pressure) in which there is usually abnormal enlargement of the ventricles and impaired contraction.

Ischemia, or impaired blood flow to the heart muscle, may also be responsible for symptoms (including chest pain) in HCM, and may have unfavorable consequences because it can cause heart cells to die and be replaced by scars (the repair process). In this regard, ischemia in HCM is similar to that experienced by patients with coronary artery disease due to atherosclerosis (with plaque in the large coronary arteries). HCM patients with ischemia may have either true angina pectoris (relatively short-lasting pain or pressure in the center of the chest associated with exertion or occurring after meals) or "atypical" pain patterns that differ from classic angina in a variety of ways.

In HCM, ischemia occurs by a different mechanism than in coronary heart disease, probably resulting from abnormal function of small arteries *within* the heart muscle which have thickened walls and narrowed openings. It is also possible that this ischemia results in part because the heart muscle is too thick for the available blood supply. Unfortunately, identifying ischemia in HCM with routinely available tests is difficult and often unreliable; positron emission tomography (PET) can be useful in this regard, but is not available for routine testing. Therefore, it has been challenging to assess this particular problem with precision in the HCM population.

Left ventricular outflow obstruction

Muscle thickening involving the upper portion of the ventricular septum is often associated with a unique motion pattern of the mitral valve. In such cases, during the ejection of the blood from the left ventricle (in systole), the mitral valve moves forward and contacts the septum (there should normally be a considerable gap between these two structures) and

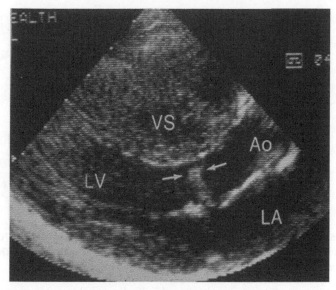

Figure 14 The unique mechanism by which obstruction occurs in HCM shown in a stop-frame echocardiogram. Note how a portion of the mitral valve comes forward to ultimately contact the thick ventricular septum (VS) (denoted by arrows). Ao, aorta; LA, left atrium; LV, left ventricle cavity.

obstructs the outflow of blood from the left side of the heart into the aorta, thereby creating a *pressure gradient* between the aorta and the left ventricle. Consequently, **left ventricular outflow obstruction** in HCM is actually caused by unique mitral valve motion and *not* due to the thickened septum, *per se* (called systolic anterior motion (SAM)) (Figure 14).

There is often considerable confusion around this point among patients, who may assume mistakenly that they have valve disease. The turbulent blood flow produced by obstruction creates a **murmur** – a sound that is audible with a stethoscope. In addition, the abnormal mitral valve motion will cause blood to leak backward into the left atrium, called **mitral regurgitation**. Together, obstruction and mitral regurgitation cause the pressures within the chamber of the left ventricle to increase, which in turn adversely affects heart function.

Outflow obstruction, although present in the resting state (such as when you are having your echocardiogram performed) in about 25% of HCM patients, also commonly occurs with physical exertion and can account (with mitral regurgitation) for symptoms such as shortness of breath, fatigue, chest pain, and fainting, which typically occur with activity. It was formerly believed that obstruction was relatively uncommon among HCM

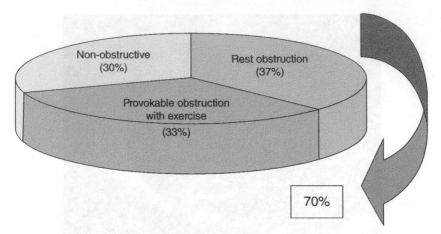

Figure 15 Obstruction to left ventricular outflow is common in HCM. About 70% of patients will have this either at rest (in the echo laboratory) or with exercise. The remaining 30% have the *nonobstructive* form of the disease.

patients because only a minority has this finding under resting conditions. However, more recent data obtained by exercising patients on the treadmill show that a large number who have no obstruction at rest do in fact develop gradients (i.e., obstruction) under normal physiologic exercise conditions. Therefore, it is now evident that 70% of all HCM patients have some obstruction either at rest or with exercise (Figure 15).

The descriptive term – *obstruction* – often conveys a strong connotation to patients which may not always be entirely deserved. This word refers, of course, to only partial obstruction (or impedance) to the flow of blood from the left ventricle to the aorta. Furthermore, the presence of obstruction is not always unfavorable to patients, and can be tolerated for many years with no or few symptoms. On the other hand, in some patients severe limiting symptoms and disability can be attributed directly to the presence of obstruction at rest or with exercise. This is the basis for performing the surgical myectomy operation (or alternatively, alcohol septal ablation).

Obstruction literally means the *difference* in pressure between the left ventricle and aorta measured in millimeters of mercury (i.e., mmHg). This measurement is now almost always made noninvasively with Doppler echocardiography, and only very rarely by invasive cardiac catheterization in which pressure measurements are made directly with catheters introduced into the heart.

It is also important for patients to realize that obstruction in HCM may change spontaneously in degree – from day to day, or hour to hour, with exercise or emotion, or even after a heavy meal or consumption of a small amount of alcohol. Therefore, patients should consider the numerical value for their gradient in light of its dynamic nature and potential change, and not necessarily as a fixed number. It is not productive to become overly concerned about the "gradient number," but nevertheless prudent to discuss with your cardiologist regarding its true significance to you.

When does HCM develop?

Since HCM is a genetic disease, the mutant gene is present from conception and all affected family members carry exactly the same mutation. While hypertrophy, as visualized with the echocardiogram, may be present at birth or in very young children, it is actually much more common for the heart to appear normal until about age 12 years in genetically affected family members. Usually hypertrophy develops in association with accelerated growth and is apparent on the echocardiogram in the teenage years by about age 12–14 years with the vast majority of patients showing significant change in muscle thickness before age 18 years. It is also possible for the heart to thicken at virtually any age. This phenomenon of "late-onset" adult hypertrophy has been observed in midlife and even beyond, but the frequency with which it occurs is unknown. Those principles are important for designing screening strategies for young HCM family members (Table 2).

Indeed, if a thickened wall becomes evident in an HCM family member on the echocardiogram during adolescence – and cannot be explained in any other way – it may be assumed to represent the mutant gene causing HCM. These changes in thickness with growth can be abrupt and striking and therefore the appearance of the heart can be altered substantially during the teenage years – that is, from completely normal (or near-normal) thickness to a very thick ventricle. HCM experts believe these changes in hypertrophy, while often alarming in appearance to the family (and even some physicians), nevertheless represent the expected ("normal") pattern in HCM dictated by the patient's DNA code by which the heart reaches its mature structural form. Therefore, the rapid growth of the heart, commonly seen in teenagers (but which can also appear at any age) does not, *per se*, represent clinical deterioration or a warning of imminent danger.

Table 2 Clinical screening strategies with echocardiography (and ECG) for detection of HCM in families*.

Age < 12 years†
- Optional unless:
  - Malignant family history of premature death from HCM, or other adverse complications
  - Competitive athlete in an intense training program
  - Onset of symptoms
  - Other clinical suspicion of early left ventricular hypertrophy

Age 12–21 years†
- Every 12–18 months

Age > 21 years
- Imaging at onset of symptoms, or possibly at 5-year intervals at least through midlife; more frequent intervals for imaging are appropriate in families with malignant clinical course, or history of late-onset HCM

---

*In family members who had not undergone genetic testing, or in whom testing was unresolved or indeterminant.
†Age range takes into consideration individual variability in achieving physical maturity, and in some patients screening may be justified at an earlier age; initial evaluation should be performed no later than early pubescence.

Moreover, the fear of many patients that their heart will continue to thicken unrestrained throughout life, ultimately resulting in a catastrophic event, is completely unfounded. In fact, in the vast majority of patients, wall thickness does not increase measurably with advancing age during adulthood (and may even decrease slightly).

Although HCM may be present for years, it is commonly diagnosed for the first time in individuals 30–40 years of age; men are recognized an average of 5 years earlier than women. However, the age at which diagnosis is first made does not necessarily indicate when HCM began, only when it has been identified; nor is age at diagnosis consistently linked to prognosis.

HCM is identified uncommonly in children and therefore is regarded as a rare disease by pediatric cardiologists. Most children diagnosed with HCM are initially suspected because of a heart murmur, transient symptoms, abnormal ECG, or family history of HCM. On occasion, this suspicion may arise during preparticipation screening for competitive athletics – with confirmation later by echocardiography.

The proportion of HCM children with important and limiting symptoms is small, and the occurrence of sudden unexpected death before age 10 years appears to be exceedingly uncommon. Nevertheless, occasionally,

HCM may be detected in young children. Most often this occurs fortuitously (by a chance occurrence) when a murmur is heard – in a healthy-appearing child, or during routine family screening. There are probably no particular long-term consequences attached to HCM should it be discovered in this way at a young age. However, when symptoms of heart failure occur very early in life, and/or hypertrophy is substantial, these findings may well connote a more severe form of the disease.

Indeed, the diagnosis of HCM in children and adolescents often represents a major dilemma for pediatric cardiologists since the patients are young and predictions regarding future prognosis are therefore much more difficult. It is possible for such circumstances to lead to overreaction and there is occasionally a tendency to pursue major interventions earlier in younger patients. On the other hand, there may also be some reluctance to initiate chronic device therapy (e.g., implantable defibrillators) because of the youthful age and healthy appearance, lack of symptoms and active lifestyle, and the likelihood of complications occurring from the device itself over many decades.

Very rarely, HCM presents during infancy with heart failure; this appears to be a particularly unfavorable development and many of these children die early despite aggressive therapy. However, of note, most infants or young children (under 4 years) with thick hearts may not have traditional HCM (with a sarcomere mutation). A number of other diverse conditions occur in this age group in which the heart manifestations can mimic HCM (most commonly Noonan syndrome and glycogen storage diseases), or rarely when diabetes is present in the mother during pregnancy – a situation in which hypertrophy of the left ventricle in the newborn quickly disappears spontaneously within a few weeks.

Gender and race

In published clinical papers, HCM is always reported to be more common in men than in women (usually about 60:40 or 65:35). However, in reality, because HCM is a genetic disease transmitted as an autosomal-dominant trait, it occurs equally in men and women. This means that HCM is *diagnosed* less frequently in women than in men but is *not less common* in women. The reason for this under-recognition in women is unresolved. However, there is evidence that women with HCM develop symptoms later in life (compared to men), are diagnosed at more advanced ages, and, in fact, experience more severe heart failure.

HCM has always been uncommonly diagnosed in African-Americans in clinical settings. Paradoxically, previously unsuspected HCM has proved to be a common cause of sudden death in young black male athletes on the athletic field. This suggests that the rarity of an HCM diagnosis in young African-Americans is probably due largely to socioeconomic factors which create more limited access to the subspecialty medical establishment (which is a prerequisite for obtaining an echocardiogram and thereby an HCM diagnosis). The distinction between HCM and "athlete's heart" can be affected by race, since slightly greater left ventricular wall thickness and certain ECG changes are normally common in African-Americans.

- HCM occurs equally in men and women.
- HCM is under-recognized in minority communities.
- Women with HCM are diagnosed less commonly, later in life, and experience symptoms later.

What are the symptoms of HCM?

It is important to realize that HCM is unusual by virtue of affecting people at virtually any age. Patients from infants (as young as the first day of life) to the elderly (as old as 90 years of age) may develop HCM-related symptoms. It is very common to have HCM and no noticeable symptoms. This sometimes creates uncertainty in patients erroneously that they may not even have HCM, because they do not "feel" it. Some patients come to recognize it in their mid-thirties or later because they feel "like they are getting old" or "slowing down." *While the absence of symptoms is obviously a favorable aspect of HCM, it does not immunize against all risks from this disease.*

Symptoms are generally similar to that of other forms of heart disease and there is no particular complaint which is unique to this disease. Most commonly, patients report symptoms of shortness of breath or chest pain. Patients often relate "good and bad days" during which symptoms may be perceived as quite different in degree. The precise basis for this variability is uncertain. However, when relating symptoms to your cardiologist, it is important not to limit your history to either extreme (i.e., the best or worst), but rather provide the complete spectrum of complaints which you experience on a daily basis. It is particularly important to advise your cardiologist of any new or consistently increased symptoms.

Shortness of breath

Exercise capacity may be limited by shortness of breath (also called exertional **dyspnea**) and fatigue. Most HCM patients experience only mild exercise limitation but occasionally it becomes severe and patients are unable to walk even one city block at a reasonable pace, or climb a flight of stairs, without stopping due to shortness of breath; a minority may experience shortness of breath at rest.

Chest pain

Chest pain or pressure (sometimes called **angina**) is a common symptom. It is usually brought on by exertion and relieved by rest, but may also occur at rest. In HCM, chest discomfort may take different forms – sharp or dull, in the center of the chest or elsewhere or prolonged and unrelated to exertion. The cause of the pain is thought to be insufficient oxygen supply to the heart muscle (**ischemia**). In HCM, the main coronary arteries are usually free of significant plaque and narrowing from atherosclerosis. However, in contrast, the small arteries within the heart muscle are often narrowed; the greatly thickened left wall ventricular muscle demands increased oxygen supply, which often cannot be served by these abnormal small arteries.

Fatigue

This is a complaint distinctive from shortness of breath with exertion; many patients complain of excessive tiredness, either related or unrelated to exertion, and the necessity to nap frequently. It is challenging to effectively treat fatigue in HCM.

Palpitations

Patients may occasionally feel an extra or skipped beat, and this may be normal and unrelated to HCM. Sometimes, however, such an awareness of the beating heart may be prolonged and indicative of an irregular heart rhythm. This symptom, **palpitations**, may also occur commonly in other heart diseases and even frequently in people without any form of heart disease. Palpitations begin suddenly, and may be associated with symptoms such as sweating or lightheadedness. Such episodes should be reported to your cardiologist and investigated.

Lightheadedness, near-fainting, and fainting

Patients with HCM may experience impairment or loss of consciousness (i.e., lightheadedness or dizziness), fainting (known as **syncope**), or the perception that loss of consciousness is imminent, but then does not, in fact, occur (**near-syncope**). Such episodes may occur in association with exercise, or without apparent provocation, and the reason for these events is not always clear, even after testing. Impaired consciousness may be due to an irregularity of the heartbeat, a fall in blood pressure, or commonly unrelated to HCM and heart disease, that is, vasovagal syncope – in which the vagal nerve is excessively active. Fainting (or near-fainting) should be reported immediately to your cardiologist and investigated. Unfortunately, such episodes represent the most difficult HCM symptom to evaluate – simply because the events occur without warning and are over long before your physician can order tests to investigate their origin.

- HCM can cause a number of symptoms including chest pain/pressure, shortness of breath, fainting/near fainting, and palpitations.
- HCM patients may not always report their symptoms – but may experience limits in endurance and stamina related to HCM.
- Sometimes it is hard to define their symptoms, as patients with HCM have lived a lifetime with this disease, making it difficult to distinguish between "normal" and "abnormal."

How is HCM diagnosed and what tests are used?

Physical examination

In many patients with HCM, the physical examination is unremarkable. Only a soft heart murmur or no murmur at all may be heard. This fact is surprising to many people, but only reflects the fact that under resting conditions most HCM patients do not have obstruction to flow of blood from the left ventricle (as discussed previously). This infrequency with which a loud heart murmur occurs accounts, in part, for the difficulty in identifying HCM during the routine preparticipation screening of competitive athletes.

Most HCM patients (particularly young people) have a prominent heart impulse that can be felt or even seen on the left side of the chest, which reflects the thickened and forcibly contracting heart. This observation may trigger suspicion of HCM in some instances, even in the absence of a loud heart murmur.

Indeed, when present, the most obvious finding on physical examination that raises suspicion of HCM is a loud systolic heart murmur. Such murmurs usually indicate partial obstruction to blood flow out of the left side of the heart, and may be transient, changing spontaneously throughout the day and with activity, or even with meals or alcohol. Your cardiologist may also be able to provoke a heart murmur by asking you to change body positions (i.e., stand) or undergo maneuvers such as holding your breath and straining (Valsalva), inhaling amyl nitrite, or exercising on a treadmill. However, in general, the presence of a heart murmur is not necessarily an unfavorable sign – it simply indicates the presence of obstruction and/or an incompetent mitral valve. While HCM may be suspected by findings on physical examination, this is usually not the way a definitive diagnosis is made.

Echocardiogram

The standard primary test for the clinical diagnosis of HCM is an ultrasound scan of the heart called a two-dimensional **echocardiogram** (Figure 16). This is an entirely safe noninvasive test which produces two-dimensional images of the heart that are viewed in real time, and recorded along with one-dimensional views (called the derived M-mode echocardiogram).

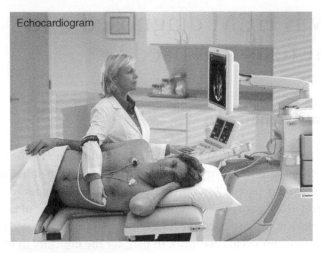

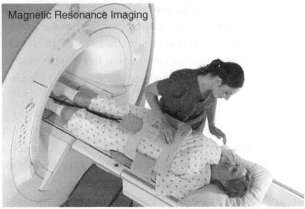

Figure 16 The clinical diagnosis of HCM is generally made with imaging tests, most commonly with an ultrasound scan of the heart called an echocardiogram (or echo, for short) (top) (image courtesy of Philips Healthcare) or alternatively (and with increasing frequency) with cardiovascular magnetic resonance (MRI or CMR) (bottom) (image courtesy of GE Medical). Both techniques are entirely safe and pain-free, and produce a number of images of the heart so that excessive thickness of the heart muscle wall (characteristic of HCM) can be easily measured. MRI has the additional capacity to visualize areas of scarring within the heart wall, and may be more reliable in identifying hypertrophy in certain regions of the left ventricle.

Echocardiograms are performed by a specially trained technologist (the cardiologist may or may not be present during the test) who places a transducer and a small amount of transmitting gel on the chest to generate images of the heart in several cross-sectional views (Figure 16). The excessive thickness of the left ventricular wall in HCM is easily (and traditionally) measured from the echocardiographic images. An additional ultrasound mode called **Doppler** is very useful with regard to heart function and includes a color-coded image of blood flow within the heart. Indeed, turbulent blood flow and the degree of obstruction (if present) as well as valve leakage (mitral regurgitation) can be detected and measured with precision.

The HCM heart usually shows thickening of the ventricular septum that exceeds that in other parts of the left ventricular wall, whether or not there is obstruction (Figure 12, Figure 17, and Figure 18). The exact pattern of hypertrophy in HCM can be quite diverse. Obstruction occurs when the mitral valve comes forward and contacts the septum during contraction, that is, the systolic anterior motion of the mitral valve known as SAM. It is not, therefore, the thick septum that is primarily responsible for obstruction, but rather the motion of the mitral valve. Therefore, the echocardiogram provides a thorough structural and functional assessment of HCM, avoiding invasive procedures such as cardiac catheterization (except under rare circumstances).

Electrocardiogram (ECG)

The standard ECG (also known as the 12-lead ECG) is performed by placing electrodes on the chest, wrists, and ankles and recording the electrical signals from the heart. In HCM, the ECG usually shows a wide variety of abnormal electrical signals usually due to the muscle thickening. Alternatively, in a minority of patients, the ECG may be normal or show only very minor alterations. The ECG abnormalities seen are not specific to HCM and may also be found in many other heart conditions. In fact, the abnormal ECG in HCM can frequently mimic that of a previous, healed, myocardial infarction ("heart attack"). Indeed, some HCM patients have been advised erroneously that they have previously experienced a "heart attack." However, keep in mind that "heart attack" is a nonmedical term which literally refers to sudden occurrences of heart damage due solely to the consequence of coronary artery disease with atherosclerosis. A potential adverse consequence of ECG patterns in HCM patients with chest pain (resembling a "heart attack") can be the inadvertent and misguided administration of nitroglycerin – otherwise contraindicated in HCM.

Cardiovascular magnetic resonance imaging (MRI or CMR)

As will be evident throughout this book, cardiovascular MRI is a contemporary imaging test, sometimes superior to echocardiography, with a number of important applications to HCM including identification of some patients at risk for sudden death (but not otherwise identifiable).

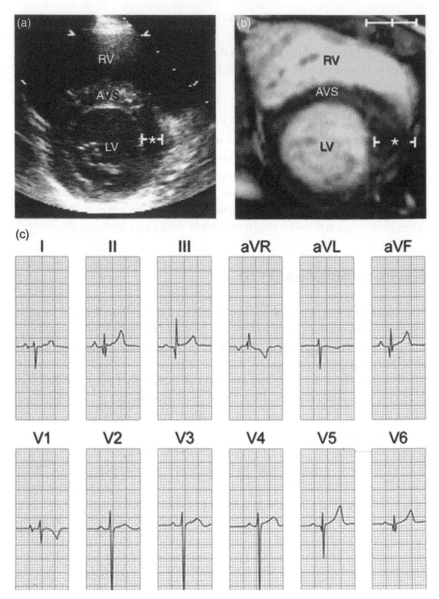

Figure 17 Capability of MRI to make the diagnosis of HCM not made by echocardiography. MRI can be superior to echocardiography in detecting hypertrophy in some areas of the left ventricle. Shown here is the MRI diagnosis in an asymptomatic 15-year-old with a family history of HCM and a distinctly abnormal ECG (as shown in (c)). (a) Normal echocardiogram. (b) MRI detects a small area of hypertrophy in a region of the left ventricle *not* reliably detected by echo (*), confirming the diagnosis of HCM. LV, left ventricle; RV, right ventricle; VS, ventricular septum.

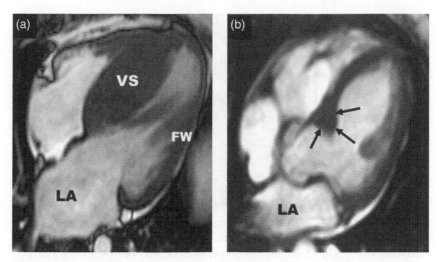

Figure 18 MRI images of HCM. (a) Markedly thick ventricular septum (VS) in contrast to the rest of the left ventricle free wall (FW). (b) Thickness of VS is limited to a small area, different from the image of the patient shown in (a), but still diagnostic of HCM. LA, left atrium.

Therefore, most HCM experts believe that MRI (with contrast) should be routinely performed in all HCM patents, probably also in the screening of family members (Figure 16, Figure 17, and Figure 18).

While two-dimensional echocardiography is the most common clinical test used to diagnose HCM, MRI has rapidly penetrated into clinical cardiology providing high-resolution images of the heart, with three-dimensional reconstruction often superior to echocardiography. MRI may allow more precise measurement of left ventricular wall thickness, including when the echocardiogram is ambiguous, or of insufficient technical quality. Notably, in selected patients, MRI may image thick areas of the wall that are inaccessible to conventional echocardiography.

Therefore, MRI may be the only imaging test capable of making the diagnosis of HCM in some patients and may also play a role in judging the level of risk for sudden death in two ways: (1) identifying areas of extreme thickening of the left ventricle which itself can be a risk factor (as discussed later); and (2) recognizing areas of scarring (Figure 19). MRI provides the opportunity to visualize scar formation (i.e., fibrosis) within the wall of the left ventricle by virtue of injecting a compound called gadolinium toward the end of the study. These areas of scar result from the death of individual heart cells and, as in the case of coronary artery disease and "heart attacks," if particularly extensive, can produce powerful arrhythmias that can predispose to sudden death.

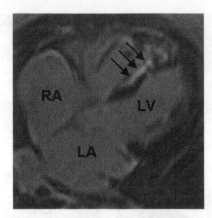

Figure 19 Scar formation in HCM. MRI with gadolinium contrast can identify scarring (arrows), appearing as white areas shown here in the septum. If extensive, such scars can be the source of important rhythm disturbances. LV, left ventricle; LA, left atrium; RA, right atrium.

However, not all patients are suitable for study with MRI, including the particularly obese and those with claustrophobia and, of course, patients with pacemakers and defibrillators, other metals, or renal compromise (excluding the administration of gadolinium).

Genetic testing

Commercial genetic testing (for genotyping HCM patients) is now widely available in the United States and several other countries. Previously, most genotyping had been through selected research laboratories. Now, in the United States, there are four fee-for-service testing laboratories (Table 1). Laboratory DNA analysis (usually 7 ml of blood) is the most definitive method for diagnosing HCM by identification of the gene mutation which is responsible for your disease. This procedure tests the known and most common genes causing HCM, as well as those conditions that mimic HCM (also known as phenocopies). Results are available in about 4–6 weeks. Expense varies considerably among the four genetic testing companies. To inquire about the cost of each provider, the Hypertrophic Cardiomyopathy Association (HCMA) website maintains a listing of each provider; as policies change from time to time, you should contact each provider to confirm fees and insurance coverage. Some companies have programs that cap the out-of-pocket expenses and others may have contracts with your individual insurance provider.

Interpretation of this test can be complex, but here is how the use of genetic testing plays out. First, knowing your mutation has no role in predicting prognosis, the clinical course of your disease, or risk of sudden death. Second, the principal value of genetic testing is in family screening – that is, in identifying family members who may be genetically affected but have a normal echocardiogram (or MRI), and may be at risk for developing the disease. Clinical screening with imaging tests is usually recommended first in order to identify those who have HCM by echocardiography and MRI.

If the option of genetic testing for family members is to proceed, this is the process (Figure 19). A family member known to have clinically expressed HCM is tested. The test result can be negative more than 50% of the time. In this case, the process ends because the family mutation has not been identified and there is nothing to act on. This occurs because there are many more genes and mutations that are not currently defined beyond the 11 genes known to cause HCM, and remarkably with about 1500 mutations. Another 25% of the time, the result is uncertain – called a "variant of unknown significance" – which means a mutation has been found, but it is not clear whether it has caused your HCM. Each human being has between 5 and 7 million mutations (variants), most of them obviously not responsible for the disease. The remaining 20–25% of time, the test identifies a mutation judged to be *pathogenic*, or responsible for HCM. This 25% is the only "actionable" situation – that is, it permits genetic screening of other family members to proceed. If another relative (such as an offspring) then tests negative for the family mutation, that individual is then designated as an unaffected member of that HCM family. If a relative without hypertrophy tests positive, they are known as "gene-positive/phenotype-negative" and are at risk for developing hypertrophy and/or disease and should be seen at annual evaluations. However, it is possible that hypertrophy will either never develop or do so many years (even decades) in the future.

- Screening for HCM in families is important and all relatives should be informed about the risk for inheritance and value of screening.
- Screening should include ECG, echocardiogram, and probably cardiac MRI conducted by a cardiologist familiar with HCM.
- Genetic testing can identify affected relatives without hypertrophy at risk for developing HCM, and can also exclude the unaffected from further screening.

Other tests that may be useful in assessing HCM in selected patients

Cardiac catheterization

Due to widespread use of noninvasive imaging with echocardiography, Doppler, and MRI, there is no longer a compelling reason to perform cardiac catheterization procedures to measure pressures or perform angiography (X-ray) to evaluate HCM. However, because it is possible for HCM patients over age 40 years (with or without a history of chest pain) to also have coronary artery disease, it may be necessary in some circumstances to perform a cardiac catheterization with angiography (X-ray) to define the anatomy of the coronary arteries due to atherosclerotic plaque. Even this role of cardiac catheterization has been reduced by the introduction of the computed tomography angiogram, which can noninvasively screen the coronary arteries for narrowings.

Electrophysiological studies

This is a specialized form of cardiac catheterization which has been performed selectively to define the risk of electrical instability, which may predispose to sudden death. *Electrophysiological studies* involve the passage of fine wires from the veins in the groin, arm, or shoulder into the heart under X-ray guidance. These wires are then used to make measurements or apply stimuli to record the response of the electrical system of the heart. Sometimes, irregularities of the heartbeat (otherwise known as **arrhythmia**) are intentionally provoked in the laboratory (and immediately terminated) to estimate a patient's predisposition to develop such rhythms naturally. At present, electrophysiological testing has been largely abandoned for assessing risk for sudden death in HCM patients.

Exercise testing

The severity of exercise limitation and the effect of treatment can be assessed with bicycle or treadmill **exercise testing**. Exercise testing can also provide an objective measurement of improvement, stability, or deterioration over time. However, a carefully taken personal history can often represent the best barometer of your physical capabilities. Of note, the exercise test is often combined with an echocardiogram (stress echocardiogram) to determine whether outflow obstruction occurs physiologically with exertion.

This particular test is used with increasing frequency on a routine basis since knowledge of such provoked obstruction may have clinical relevance, that is, to replicate the circumstances under which patients typically experience exertion-related symptoms.

If you have limiting shortness of breath, but no obstruction at rest, your cardiologist may want to perform a stress echocardiogram to determine whether you develop obstruction while engaged in physical activity which produces symptoms. This may allow you to become a candidate for a potentially beneficial treatment intervention such as surgical myectomy, or alcohol septal ablation (in selected patients). In addition, blood pressure drop or its failure to increase appropriately during exercise in some patients may indicate an important instability, and currently is a potential risk factor for sudden death.

Ambulatory ECG monitoring

The Holter ECG test is a noninvasive and continuous recording of the heartbeat over 24 or 48 hours during normal ambulatory activities. A Holter monitor is a simple test that will detect potentially important irregularities of the heartbeat which the patient is usually unaware of and is accompanied by a diary (log) to record symptoms. Longer-term monitoring for several weeks is now possible, as is the capability to transmit data via wireless technology.

Radionuclide studies

In these tests, substances producing very tiny (safe) amounts of radioactivity are injected into the bloodstream to create a heart scan. These tests are occasionally performed in HCM patients to assess the contraction capability and filling of the ventricles, at rest and with exercise.

Inaccurate diagnosis

The HCMA has systematically assembled specific clinical information from about 5000 families with HCM. It is apparent that failure to reliably diagnose HCM is linked to age, gender, and geography. In our informal survey of 1626 HCM respondents, patients had been initially diagnosed with a condition *other than* HCM (sometimes with very long periods of time before the correct diagnosis emerged). For example, children and adolescents may be incorrectly diagnosed with asthma (frequently "exercise-induced asthma"), particularly in athletes. This is of concern as some asthma medications (mainly albuterol-containing inhalers) contain properties that may promote arrhythmias in HCM. "Innocent heart murmur" is also a particularly common first diagnosis.

Men with HCM may be told they have "athlete's heart" when in fact their symptoms are directly linked to HCM. Both men and women are frequently labeled with depression. While depression and panic disorders are important diagnoses, it is possible to have these conditions as well as HCM. Women with HCM are often initially diagnosed with mitral valve prolapse or panic disorders. Patients with HCM living in rural areas appear to be diagnosed later, and face longer periods of ambiguity, than those living in urban areas. Minorities, particularly African-Americans, are underdiagnosed with HCM.

General outlook for patients with HCM

The severity of symptoms and risk of complications vary greatly between HCM patients, and it should be emphasized that many individuals never experience serious problems related to their disease. Indeed, HCM may not reduce life expectancy and is compatible with normal longevity. It is not unusual for patients to be in their 70s and 80s, including even some patients who have survived into their 90s, without significant disability, impaired quality of life, or the requirement for major treatment interventions to achieve these goals. When considering the *overall* adult population with HCM, this disease may not add significantly to individual risk – over the known risks of living, such as those related to cancer, diabetes, coronary heart disease, accidents, or other causes (Figure 20 and Figure 21). The most accurate mortality rate characterizing the overall disease is about 1% per year, which means that each year no more than 1 of 100 patients with HCM may die for any reason (not necessarily limited to HCM). This is the same expectation as for the general population of the same age.

On the other hand, many patients experience symptoms such as shortness of breath, chest pain, dizziness, or fainting, usually exertion-related, with this disability often variable from day to day ("good" and "bad" days). Although relatively uncommon, there are three circumstances in which patients with HCM may die prematurely: (1) suddenly and unexpectedly, most commonly younger patients less than 40 years of age; (2) related to severe progressive heart failure, usually in midlife; and (3) due to stroke, generally in older patients with atrial fibrillation. Limiting symptoms (i.e., shortness of breath and/or chest pain with exertion) may remain stable and controlled with treatment for many years or deteriorate and require additional therapeutic intervention. However, each patient with HCM

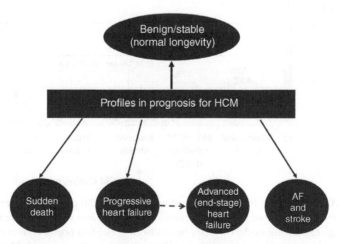

Figure 20 Profiles in prognosis. Most patients with HCM can be placed in one of these pathways for the purpose of judging prognosis, and eventually formulating treatment strategies. This diagram emphasizes the necessity of viewing HCM in terms of such subgroups so that treatment can be tailored to a particular clinical profile. However, notably not all patients experience disease complications, and many enjoy a benign and stable course. AF, atrial fibrillation.

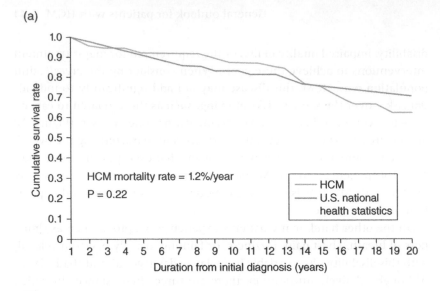

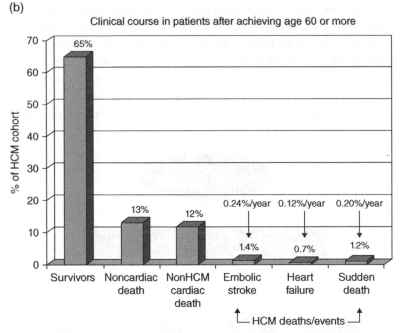

Figure 21 Survival with HCM. (a) Survival in a regional HCM population from the upper-West compared to that in the general US population (mortality due to all causes; e.g., cancer, homicide, coronary heart disease). The two populations are not different in terms of survival (mortality risk for both is about 1% per year). Therefore, HCM itself does not add to the overall risk of living. (b) Aging and survival with HCM to age 60 or more appears to be associated with a low subsequent sudden death rate of only 0.2%/year, lower than the risk in the general population. Therefore, the risk for sudden death appears to generally *decrease* after 60 years.

must be assessed individually to determine which subgroup of patients they most likely belong to – for example, high or low risk for sudden death, with or without predisposition to progressive symptoms, or with or without atrial fibrillation (Figure 20).

Therefore, an important general principle regarding HCM is that all patients are *not* the same in terms of prognosis, clinical presentation, or potential treatment options. *One treatment does not fit all in HCM* (Figure 20). Since there are several different clinical profiles that patients may adopt, it is important not to "lump" all patients together under one homogeneous label of HCM. Indeed, while some patients have little or no risk associated with their disease, others deserve high-risk status. *However, the overall disease is not, per se, high risk, and HCM should not be regarded as a uniformly unfavorable condition.* Obviously, this book provides only a broad overview of prognosis for HCM patients and cannot substitute for the careful evaluation of an individual patient by a cardiologist knowledgeable about this disease, particularly one in a HCM center.

Complications of HCM

Arrhythmias

A variety of arrhythmias (irregularities of the heartbeat) are exceedingly common in patients with HCM and can be detected by Holter monitoring, exercise testing, or ECG (Figure 20 and Figure 28). Prolonged arrhythmias known as **ventricular tachycardia** or **atrial fibrillation** are particularly important and require treatment in the vast majority of cases. Transient arrhythmias with premature beats originating from the atria and ventricles occur much more commonly, but usually do not have particular clinical importance to HCM patients, even when present in large numbers.

Ventricular tachycardia/ventricular fibrillation
Ventricular tachycardia is an incessant and repetitive occurrence of abnormal beats arising from the ventricles. This is a potentially serious arrhythmia in HCM since it may lead to ventricular fibrillation and sudden death. Selected patients prone to these arrhythmias may be treated with an

implantable cardioverter defibrillator, designed to sense and automatically terminate these arrhythmias (as will be discussed later).

Atrial fibrillation and stroke

With atrial fibrillation, the normal regular heart rhythm is altered due to loss of the contraction of the atria (the two upper chambers), causing the ventricles to beat in an irregular rhythm. Atrial fibrillation may be episodic (i.e., paroxysmal) or persistent (i.e., chronic), occurs in as many as 20–25% of HCM patients (about four times more common than in the general population), and is often responsible for important symptoms of heart failure, but does not appear to be specifically associated with increased risk for sudden unexpected death. While some patients are unaware of their atrial fibrillation, most will rapidly develop symptoms such as shortness of breath and rapid heart rate, dizziness, and fainting, or more nonspecific sensations of "not feeling right." Atrial fibrillation increases in frequency with age, but may occur at any time in adulthood (usually after age 30–35). Atrial fibrillation is much less common in younger patients, and is exceedingly rare in children. Enlargement of the left atrium appears to predispose to atrial fibrillation.

Because the atria "fibrillate" there is risk for clot formation due to stagnant blood flow. This can result in a stroke if the blood clot travels to the brain. The risk of such an event is about 1% per year in HCM patients with atrial fibrillation. However, anticoagulation, to protect against stroke, is an important consideration, and the pros and cons of this treatment should be discussed in detail with your cardiologist.

Sometimes atrial fibrillation will revert to normal rhythm or control and reduce the rapid heart rate from the ventricles (if the patient must remain in atrial fibrillation). However, **electrical cardioversion** may be used to convert the heart back into its normal rhythm. This treatment requires admission to the hospital and consists of applying an electrical shock to the chest, often following a course of anticoagulant medication. Atrial fibrillation also occurs in other non-HCM heart diseases (as well as in patients without heart disease – i.e., "lone atrial fibrillation").

Other treatments for atrial fibrillation in HCM include the MAZE procedure, in which the electrical connection in the left atria is interrupted at surgery, and is sometimes performed with myectomy. Also, radiofrequency ablation is a novel nonsurgical procedure in which energy is delivered through the tip of a catheter interrupting the abnormal electrical pathways. This treatment is also sometimes referred to as pulmonary vein isolation since the focus for atrial fibrillation is usually in the pulmonary vein (and not left atrium proper). This procedure is being performed more frequently with increasing success (and with lessening complications) in HCM patients with frequent episodes of paroxysmal atrial fibrillation, which impairs quality of life.

- Approximately 20% of HCM patients will experience atrial fibrillation (or atrial flutter) at some time.
- Atrial fibrillation usually requires anticoagulation therapy.
- Radiofrequency ablation may become a means of reducing or eliminating atrial fibrillation in HCM.

Heart failure

HCM patients with significant shortness of breath during physical exertion are, strictly speaking, experiencing a degree of heart failure. However, this is a different form of heart failure than occurs in patients with coronary artery disease, or other cardiac conditions. Usually in HCM, heart failure is paradoxically present in a heart in which the ventricles are not dilated and show normal contraction. In other more common diseases, congestive heart failure can be a profound and chronic condition, generally occurring after a myocardial infarction ("heart attack"), and producing enlarged or dilated ventricles that contract poorly. Occasionally, heart failure in HCM may become intractable and fail to respond to drugs, requiring major intervention and treatment, such as with surgical myectomy (alcohol septal ablation as a selective alternative).

- Heart failure, although ominous sounding, means only that you are short of breath with exertion.
- Mild transient symptoms are common.
- Many (if not most) patients will not experience heart failure.
- Severe heart failure may require major treatment intervention, although this is rare among all patients.

The problem of sudden death

Since the first description of HCM more than 50 years ago, the issue of risk for sudden and unexpected death has been a highly visible issue (Figure 20, Figure 21, Figure 22, Figure 23, Figure 24, Figure 25, Figure 26,

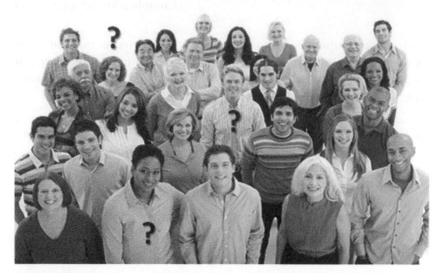

Figure 22 While the risk for sudden death in young people has been a highly visible feature of HCM, in reality it is an uncommon occurrence and only a minority of patients are truly at risk. Therefore, an important aspiration of the HCM evaluation is to identify which specific patients, among all those with this condition, are at unacceptably high risk.

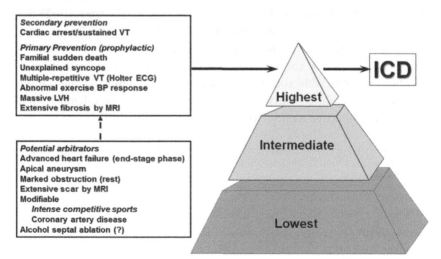

Figure 23 Assessing risk in HCM. There are a number of disease features that can (in the judgment of your cardiologist) raise the perceived risk for sudden death and place an individual patient in the top part of the risk pyramid where an ICD can be discussed and considered. Secondary prevention means an ICD is placed after surviving a cardiac arrest, and there is no dispute in the cardiology community over this decision. Primary prevention means the decision to implant an ICD prophylactically, based on the risk factors shown in the box. The presence of one or more of these risk markers may be sufficient to assign high-risk status and justify consideration for an ICD. "Arbitrators" are disease features that may resolve borderline ICD decisions. BP, blood pressure; LVH, left ventricular hypertrophy; VT, ventricular tachycardia.

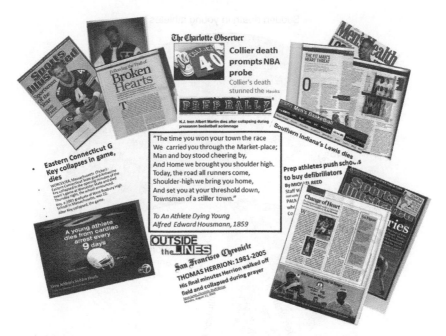

Figure 24 Athletic field deaths in young sports participants have achieved a high level of public visibility in the news media. HCM is the single most common cause of these deaths. A 117-year-old poem which reflects the public perception of athlete sudden deaths then, which is true even to this day.

and Figure 27). However, it should be emphasized that in reality only a small proportion of patients with HCM are at increased risk for sudden premature death due to arrhythmias. Also, the magnitude of this problem of sudden death has probably been exaggerated over the years due to the disproportionate number of reports from institutions in which there was a preferential referral of high-risk patients (i.e., the tertiary referral centers) and media attention to HCM as the cause of sudden death in trained athletes.

The reality is that only a very small fraction of all HCM patients are at risk to die suddenly. Nevertheless, understandingly, sudden unexpected collapse remains a devastating consideration for many patients living with this disease. Unfortunately, there are no reliable clinical warning signs and the assignment of high-risk status is not dependent on the prior occurrence of symptoms. Therefore, the absence of symptoms can represent a false sense of security for patients with respect to sudden death risk.

We know that sudden death occurs most commonly in young people (under 30–35 years old), but on the other hand there is no particular age

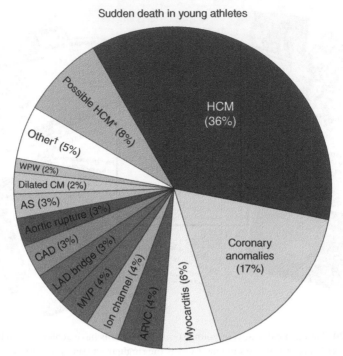

Sudden death in young athletes

- HCM (36%)
- Coronary anomalies (17%)
- Possible HCM* (8%)
- Other† (5%)
- WPW (2%)
- Dilated CM (2%)
- AS (3%)
- Aortic rupture (3%)
- CAD (3%)
- LAD bridge (3%)
- MVP (4%)
- Ion channel (4%)
- ARVC (4%)
- Myocarditis (6%)

Figure 25 Sudden death in young trained athletes. HCM accounts for about one-third of these tragic events. Several other (mostly congenital) forms of heart disease shown here are less commonly responsible for deaths in young athletes. ARVC, arrhythmogenic right ventricular cardiomyopathy; AS, aortic stenosis; CAD, coronary artery disease (due to atherosclerosis); CHD, congenital heart disease; CM, cardiomyopathy; LAD, left anterior descending coronary artery; LVH, left ventricular hypertrophy; MVP, mitral valve prolapse; WPW, Wolff–Parkinson–White.

which is completely immune, and these events have not uncommonly been reported in midlife. The first 10–12 years of life are generally, but not invariably, free of adverse events (at a time when it is also uncommon for hypertrophy to appear). Only a few early-onset cases of young children with substantial hypertrophy or sudden death have been reported.

Sudden death occurs in some susceptible patients with HCM probably because the abnormal heart muscle can sometimes interfere with normal electrical activity (i.e., cause electrical instability). For example, in those portions of the left ventricular wall with abnormal architecture and cell disarray, the electrical signal may become unstable as it crosses areas of scarring and disorganized cells (Figure 1 and Figure 12). This can, in turn, lead to distorted electrical impulses that generate fast or erratic heart rhythms, some of which can result in adverse clinical events.

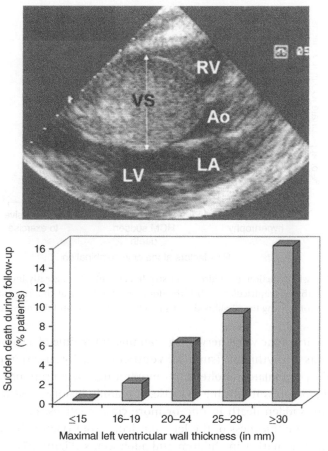

Figure 26 Extreme thickening matters in HCM. (Top) A stop-frame photograph from a two-dimensional echocardiogram of an HCM heart in which the thickness of the ventricular septum (VS) is about five times the normal. Ao = aorta; LA = left atrium; LV = left ventricle; RV = right ventricle. (Bottom) Population study showing that there is little risk for sudden death associated with mild degrees of thickening of the left ventricular wall, while extreme wall thickening of 30 mm or more conveys the highest risk, and can be a reason for your cardiologist to recommend an ICD. VP, mitral valve prolapse; WPW, Wolff–Parkinson–White. (Source: Spirito P et al, NEJM 2000;324:1778–1785. Reproduced with permission of Massachusetts Medical Society)

A patient's risk for sudden death is judged by the presence or absence of certain disease features or events. At present, the highest risk for sudden death appears to be associated with the following (Figure 23): (1) prior cardiac arrest (complete heart stoppage); (2) fainting, particularly when associated with exertion and in young people, and *not* when due to

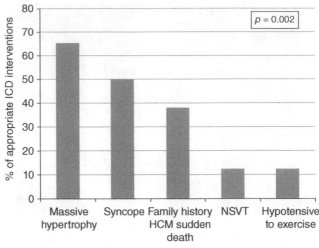

Figure 27 Risk prediction in children. Massive hypertrophy (i.e., greatly increased thickness of the left ventricular wall) is the dominant risk factor in children and adolescents for judging the likelihood of a sudden death event, and the need for an ICD.

hyperactivity of the vagal nerve (e.g., fainting at the time of a blood draw); (3) serious arrhythmias (such as ventricular tachycardia) repeatedly detected by ambulatory Holter ECG monitoring; (4) a drop, or failure to rise, of blood pressure during exercise; (5) family history of HCM-related premature sudden death in one or more close relatives; or (6) extreme increase in the thickness of the left ventricular wall (Figure 26) the most important risk marker in children and adolescents (Figure 27). The latter disease feature applies to HCM patients in whom the maximum thickness of the left ventricular wall is 3.0 cm (30 mm) or more, and who, therefore, may be at increased risk based solely on their particular heart structure.

There are a number of new perspectives on sudden death risk that deserve emphasis. First, it is now evident that *age* plays a role in the level of risk that we had not previously anticipated – that is, older age (>60 years) is associated with *lower risk* (an "antirisk factor" in a sense) (Figure 21). That means, in general, that stable HCM patients in the seventh decade without symptoms likely have a disease that has declared itself to be more benign, even if risk markers are present. Therefore, a 65-year-old patient with one or more risk factors is likely not at the same level of risk as a 25-year-old with exactly the same clinical profile, and consideration for a prophylactic implantable cardioverter defibrillator (ICD) in that 65-year-old patient is much reduced.

Second, due to a recent interest in MRIs for HCM, it has now become evident that this test when combined with a contrast agent called *gadolinium* may be used to detect scars (a form of heart damage resulting from the death of heart cells). When this scarring is *extensive* (but *only* when extensive), it may represent a new marker for sudden death, even when other more conventional risk factors are absent.

In this regard, the term "risk stratification" is used to describe those tests, symptoms, and disease characteristics which are conventionally used to determine whether a given patient should be regarded at "high risk" or increased risk for sudden cardiac arrest (SCA) (Figure 23). Patients with one or more major risk factors are encouraged to discuss ICD therapy with their cardiologist. Unfortunately, we know that occasionally patients with none of the known risk factors may also suffer cardiac arrest. At present, until further research clarifies this issue, assignment to the low-risk category is not an absolute 100% guarantee. Therefore, it is an unfortunate fact that in HCM (as in other cardiac diseases) a small number of patients without evidence of risk (and ineligible for ICDs) may nevertheless be at risk.

On the other hand, and deserving of equal emphasis, the vast majority of HCM patients without sudden death risk factors are, in fact, at low risk for premature death, and therefore are deserving of a large measure of reassurance in this regard. Although HCM patients have a life expectancy generally similar to the overall US population (Figure 21), the level of risk can change over time, and therefore risk stratification should be performed every 1–2 years. This is only one of the justifications for regular surveillance in this disease.

- Sudden death risk assessment is important.
- Risk assessment must be revisited on a systematic basis as clinical profile can change and our understanding of risk factors change.
- Revisiting risk is one of the justifications for annual visits and surveillance by your cardiologist.
- Having no risk factors is not an absolute guarantee against the very small possibility of sudden death.

Endocarditis

Endocarditis is an infection of the heart which occurs very uncommonly in HCM. Nevertheless, it is important to be protected from the unlikely disease complication since severe tissue damage of the heart valve can result, sometimes necessitating surgical replacement. Bacteria which gain access to the bloodstream can stick to the inside of the heart (specifically on the mitral valve) after it has been roughened by turbulent blood flow. The risk of bacterial endocarditis in HCM seems to be largely limited to those with obstruction, which we now know is present in 70% of all patients either at rest or with exercise.

Aneurysms in HCM

A small proportion of HCM patients (about 1–2%) may develop a relatively small area of the left ventricle at its tip in which the wall bulges outward due to thinning and scarring. Aneurysms are important because they can be the source of serious arrhythmias, and may justify placement of an implantable defibrillator to prevent sudden death (if this is the judgment of your cardiologist). However, there is no evidence at present that these aneurysms can rupture, and there is also little information available regarding whether they enlarge and, if so, at what rate. Aneurysms are identified best with MRI, which can also show the scarring within the rim of the aneurysm and beyond in surrounding areas of the left ventricle. If large, the aneurysm can be seen with echocardiography, but MRI is the most reliable test for identifying all sizes, which explains why these aneurysms in HCM patients remained "undiscovered" for so long. The mechanism by which these aneurysms form in HCM is unknown.

Advanced heart failure ("end-stage" phase)

This part of the HCM disease spectrum is also discussed later in more detail within the section on heart transplantation, to which it is linked clinically. The "end-stage" is characterized by a change in the structure and function of the left ventricle due to a gradual scarring process (which is not reversible), and ultimately results in impaired contractility and enlargement of the cavity and progressive heart failure.

- Patients may experience none, or one, or more of the HCM complications.
- HCM has a multitude of treatment options to address each potential complication.
- Family members generally experience differing clinical courses.

Special considerations: athletes and sports activities

While sudden death is very uncommon among all HCM patients, HCM is nevertheless the most frequent cause of sudden cardiac death in young people, including participants in organized and sanctioned high school and college competitive sports (Figure 24 and Figure 25). While HCM is responsible for one-third of such deaths, several (about 20) other congenital or genetic disorders can also result in such catastrophes. In HCM, the mechanism by which sudden death occurs is a ventricular arrhythmia (rhythm disturbance), in some way triggered by the intense physical activity itself. Based on these observations, it has been prudent to withdraw young people from intense competitive sports when the diagnosis of HCM is made in order to lower their risk. It should be emphasized that systematic participation in intense competitive sports can itself represent a sudden death risk marker, even in the absence of all other evidence of risk related to the disease itself. This applies to most organized athletic activities, particularly those involving exertion during which heart rate increases abruptly. Alternatively, participation in a few low-intensity competitive sports, such as golf and bowling, are more acceptable. It is largely accepted that competitive athletics, or any lifestyle consistently involving physical exertion, adds to the risk of serious consequences from HCM – and removal from such activities will restore that individual to a more acceptable risk level. Indeed, removal of athletes with HCM from organized competitive sports can itself be regarded as a potentially beneficial treatment strategy. When the HCM diagnosis is made early in life, it can be regarded as an opportunity to steer that young patient away from engagement in competitive athletics in advance.

National recommendations concerning criteria for competitive sports eligibility and disqualification with cardiovascular disease have been formalized in a document known as *Bethesda Conference #36*, sponsored by the American College of Cardiology and published in the *Journal of the American College of Cardiology* in 2005.

Young patients with HCM often wish to exercise and participate in *recreational* physical activities, whether or not they have personally been active in competitive sports. Such recommendations are often complex. However, an American Heart Association document is available providing

specific guidelines for HCM and recreational sports (Table 3). These guidelines recommend avoiding recreational sports activities that involve
1 "Burst" (sprinting) exertion with rapid acceleration and deceleration (and not abrupt change in heart rate) over short distances.
2 Adverse environmental conditions including particularly cold or hot (and humid) temperatures.
3 Systematic and progressive levels of exertion and training focused on achieving higher levels of conditioning and excellence.
4 Excessive or prolonged participation in sports otherwise intended to be recreational and moderate.

Table 3 Recommendations regarding physical activity and recreational (noncompetitive) sports participation for young patients with clinical diagnosis of HCM.

Sport	Level of exercise (Eligibility)	Sport	Level of exercise (Eligibility)
Basketball		Motorcycling	3
Full court	0	Jogging	3
Half court	0	Sailing[†]	3
Body building*	1	Surfing[†]	2
Ice Hockey*	0	Swimming (lap)*	5
Gymnastics	2	Tennis (doubles)	4
Racquetball/squash	0	Treadmill/stationary bicycle	5
Rock climbing*	1	Weightlifting (free weights)*[§]	1
Running (sprinting)	0	Hiking	3
Skiing (downhill)*	2	Bowling	5
Skiing (cross country)	2	Golf	5
Soccer	0	Horseback riding*	3
Tennis (singles)	0	Scuba diving[†]	0
Touch (flag) football	1	Skating (nonhockey)	5
Windsurfing[†]	1	Snorkeling[†]	5
Baseball/softball	2	Weights (nonfree weights)	4
Biking	4	Brisk walking	5
Modest hiking	4		

Reproduced with permission of American Heart Association from Maron BJ et al., Circulation 2004;109:2807–2816.
Recreational sports are graded on a relative scale (0–5) for eligibility, with 0–1 indicating generally not advised or strongly discouraged; 4–5 indicating probably permitted; and 2–3 indicating intermediate (and to be assessed clinically on an individual patient basis).
*These sports involve the potential for traumatic injury, which should be taken into consideration for patients with a risk for impaired consciousness.
†The possibility of syncope occurring during water-related activities should be taken into account with respect to the clinical profile of the individual patient.
§Recommendations are generally more flexible for the use of weight-training machines (i.e., nonfree weights).

Not uncommonly, healthy trained athletes (without HCM) have hypertrophy of the left ventricle (i.e., mild thickening of the wall) that results from intense and prolonged athletic training, and which may resemble HCM. This thickening is referred to as "physiologic" to separate it as the "normal" process stimulated by training in athletes ("athlete's heart"). Clinical distinctions between the two diagnoses can be difficult in some individuals, but can often be resolved with noninvasive testing (i.e., echocardiography, MRI, and, in some cases, genetic testing). This is obviously an important distinction since HCM is a disease with potentially adverse consequences, while the changes in heart structure produced only by athletic training (i.e., "athlete's heart) are not believed to have any important clinical implications to patients.

- HCM is the leading cause of SCA in the young, including competitive athletes.
- HCM is not compatible with intense competitive sports.
- Children, adolescents, and young adults may require considerable support while transitioning to a life without competitive sports.

Treatments for HCM

There are several treatment options available directed toward improving heart function, relieving symptoms, and preventing the complications of HCM such as sudden death. Patients with no symptoms may not require treatment, unless they are judged to be at increased risk for sudden death. For patients who require therapy for their disease, one or more of the following strategies may be considered (Figure 28).

Medical management

Medications are usually the first line of treatment for HCM patients experiencing heart failure symptoms of shortness of breath and chest pain associated with exertion, and many patients benefit from the administration of such medications with a reduction in those symptoms. A relatively small number of drugs are currently used in treating HCM, and the choice of

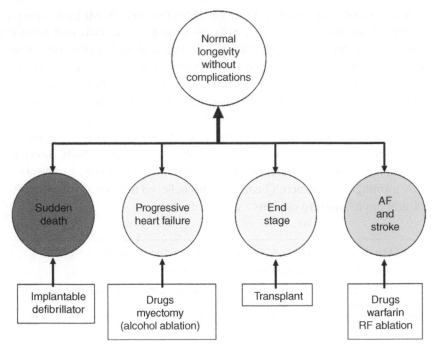

Figure 28 HCM is a contemporary treatable disease. Each of the disease complications has effective treatment strategies. Many patients do not incur serious consequences from HCM, do not evolve along these pathways, and do not require major treatments. AF, atrial fibrillation.

which one to use first is often made on an individual patient basis. When children with HCM develop such symptoms, they are treated with the same drugs, but in reduced dosage. The drugs most commonly used in HCM are described in the following list.

Beta-blockers

These are popular cardiovascular medications. There are approximately 20 different beta-blocking drugs available worldwide. Beta-blockers slow the heart rate, reduce the force of contraction, probably improve filling of the ventricles in diastole, decrease the oxygen demand of the heart, and can also be administered to decrease obstruction provoked during exercise. Beta-blockers are also widely used in medical practice for the treatment of other types of heart disease, including high blood pressure and heart failure following a heart attack, or other cardiomyopathies. However, sometimes, beta-blockers can produce excessive fatigue, lightheadedness, nightmares, and occasionally impotence. But all these side effects are reversible once the drug is withdrawn. Several beta-blockers are available for use in HCM: propranolol (Inderal®), atenolol (Tenormin®), nadolol (Corgard®), and metoprolol (Lopressor®; Toprol XL®). Long-acting preparations of these drugs, requiring only a single daily dosage, are now used predominantly. Termination of beta-blockers should occur by reducing the dose of the drug gradually over a week. It is not advisable to suddenly stop taking a beta-blocker because of the chance that your shortness of breath and/or chest pain may come back suddenly. Always consult your cardiologist prior to discontinuing any medications used in HCM.

- Beta-blockers are usually the first-line drug treatment when symptoms arise.
- Other drugs are available: verapamil, as well as disopyramide and diuretics.
- Medication may start at a low dose and be increased as symptoms warrant.
- There are several drugs that should be avoided in most patients with HCM.

Calcium channel blockers

The second major group of drugs is calcium channel blockers, with verapamil (Calan®; Isoptin®) being the most commonly administered to HCM patients. This drug appears to relax the heart and improve filling of the ventricles (during diastole). In addition, liked beta-blockers, verapamil can cause slowing of the heart rate and lower blood pressure; some patients also experience constipation, dizziness, and ankle edema. However, other calcium antagonists such as nifedipine (Procardia-XL®), and also angiotensin-converting enzyme (ACE) inhibitor drugs, should be avoided because of the risk of provoking outflow obstruction. Beta-blockers and verapamil are usually not administered together because this combination may lower the heart rate and/or blood pressure excessively. Another calcium blocker, diltiazem (Cardizem®; Dilacore-XL®), has also been used occasionally in HCM, but there are few data on its efficacy specifically in this disease.

Disopyramide (Norpace®)

This is a drug which relaxes the heart and is also an antiarrhythmic agent. Disopyramide has been used less commonly than beta-blockers and verapamil to treat HCM patients with symptoms. Nevertheless, disopyramide (which is usually administered with a beta-blocker) is unique among HCM drugs, as it is the only one with the capability to decrease obstruction at rest to some degree. Importantly, disopyramide apparently has little propensity to provoke arrhythmias in HCM. Of note, when patients become severely limited despite maximal drug treatment due to obstruction, it is unlikely that continued medical therapy (or further increases in dosages) will reduce symptoms substantially at that point in the clinical course, and it is best to consider reversing heart failure with surgery (or, alternatively, with alcohol ablation in selected patients).

Amiodarone (Cordarone®; Pacerone®)

This drug is used in HCM, usually to reduce the chances of recurrent episodes of atrial fibrillation. However, notably, amiodarone does have several potentially important side effects. The most important of these is lung fibrosis (which may not be reversible), altered thyroid function (particularly hypothyroidism), and sensitivity to ultraviolet (UV) sunlight with blue-gray discoloration of the skin (which may be largely reversible). The latter side effect may be prevented by sunblock barrier creams.

For these reasons, it is always uncertain whether amiodarone can be tolerated for particularly long periods of time in individual patients, particularly young people at high risk for sudden death. This is one of the reasons amiodarone has been abandoned as a primary treatment for high-risk HCM patients who may be susceptible to ventricular tachycardia fibrillation and sudden death. Some cardiologists have used the antiarrhythmic drug *sotolol* (Betapace®), which combines some of the properties of amiodarone and a beta-blocker, but there are virtually no data for HCM patients. Other antiarrhythmic drugs such as quinidine and procainamide have been abandoned due to their propensity to paradoxically induce important arrhythmias. A new alternative to amiodarone for the control of atrial fibrillation is dronedarone (Multaq®).

Diuretics

Most patients with HCM do not require diuretics (water tablets) for management of their symptoms. However, some severely symptomatic patients develop fluid retention, and in that situation diuretics, which increase urine flow, may be administered judiciously. The most common diuretics are furosemide (Lasix®), hydrochlorothiazide (HCTZ), and a combination of HCTZ and triamterene (Dyazide®, Maxzide®). Even though diuretics often eliminate fluid buildup in the lungs and in the extremities, these drugs should be taken with caution in HCM patients for two reasons. First of all, dehydration may result, which could lead to an increase in obstruction and symptoms. Second, diuretics tend to cause electrolyte (potassium, magnesium, calcium) depletion, which may predispose to dangerous arrhythmias. Therefore, patients who take diuretics are often checked by their physician for electrolyte deficiency (such as potassium) and are prescribed electrolyte supplementation in tablet forms.

Anticoagulants

Most patients with episodic or persistent atrial fibrillation should take anticoagulants ("blood thinners," usually Coumadin® (warfarin)) to prevent stroke, which may result if a clot forms due to stasis of blood in the atria, and a portion breaks off and travels through the arterial bloodstream to the brain. Such treatment requires monitoring with a blood test (called international normalized ratio (INR)), approximately on a monthly basis. Given the potential complications of anticoagulation (e.g., hemorrhage from trauma), the decision of whether to begin anticoagulation treatment may be a difficult one and obviously should be made in close consultation with your cardiologist.

Prodaxa® (Dabigatran) is a new drug used in atrial fibrillation to protect against stroke, as a direct thrombin inhibitor (i.e., reduces the ability of thrombin to cause clots). This drug has the advantage of avoiding monitoring, but is not recommended for the elderly and those with kidney problems.

Drugs to be avoided

Conversely, there are some drugs which generally should be avoided in HCM. For example, medications which dilate peripheral vessels such as nitroglycerin, ACE inhibitors (lisinopril, ramipril), and angiotensin-receptor blockers (losartan and others) are not usually prescribed to patients with HCM because of their ability to potentially promote obstruction. Digoxin (digitalis) is usually avoided as it increases the strength and vigor of heart contractions, but can be useful in the treatment of systolic heart failure ("end-stage" HCM). Many noncardiac medications should be avoided (or taken only after consultation with your physician) including those that manage and control migraine headaches, asthma, and allergy or any drug that can excessively vasodilate (open veins to increase blood flow) or stimulate increased heart rate.

Antibiotics

Although **endocarditis** is rare in HCM, patients with obstruction either at rest or with exercise (in which there is turbulent blood flow in the left ventricle) should receive **antibiotic prophylaxis** prior to any dental procedures (including cleaning), as well as other surgical interventions to prevent **bacterial endocarditis** (literally, an infection of the heart).

Of note, the most recent American Heart Association recommendations do not advise antibiotics to prevent bacterial endocarditis in HCM. However, all HCM experts and the HCMA regard this as a colossal mistake, imprudent and not in the best interest of HCM patients. Therefore, it is recommended to continue with the *old* American Heart Association (AHA) guidelines and arrange for antibiotic prophylaxis with your dentist at the time your dental appointment is made, well in advance of the procedure.

Implantable defibrillators

HCM patients clearly at high risk for sudden death may be candidates for an **ICD**, a sophisticated device which is permanently implanted internally and is capable of sensing potentially lethal arrhythmias and then automatically introducing a shock to terminate these arrhythmias and restore normal heart rhythm for preservation of life (Figure 29, Figure 30, Figure 31, Figure 32, and Figure 33). At the same time, an ECG recording is stored in the device to permit documentation of the event.

Over the past decade, there has been increasing experience with (and interest in) employing ICD therapy in high-risk patients with genetic heart diseases (such as HCM), including some children. The ICD represents a major innovation, as it is capable of favorably changing the clinical course of HCM for many patients by preventing sudden death, and indeed is the only treatment in HCM proven to prolong life.

In the largest study published to date, ICD appropriately intervened, aborting potentially lethal arrhythmias in individually high-risk patients at a rate of 5% per year. This rate of discharge was highest if the ICD was placed because of a prior cardiac arrest (11% per year), but was also substantial in those patients for whom the device was implanted for one or more of the HCM risk factors and without a prior major clinical event (about 4% per year). Most of those patients for whom the ICD is life-saving are young and without significant symptoms. Similar findings have been reported in children and adolescents with ICDs implanted before age 20.

ICDs have become smaller and much easier to implant in unobtrusive positions on the chest, requiring in most instances only an overnight hospital stay without major surgery. The generator (containing the battery) is now, on average, $2 \times 3 \times 1/2$ inches and fits just below the clavicle, the usual site of implant. ICD leads are introduced into the heart chamber through the veins.

(a)

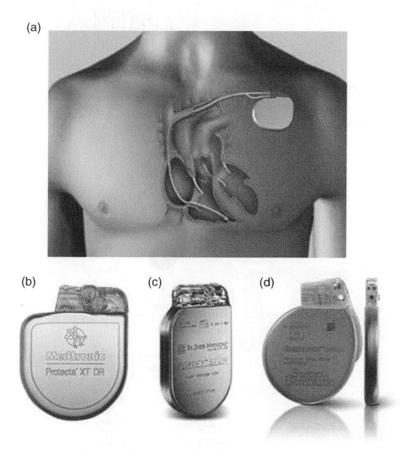

(b)   (c)   (d)

Figure 29 The implantable cardioverter defibrillator (ICD). HCM patients judged to be at high risk can be permanently implanted with a device that automatically detects and terminates life-threatening arrhythmias. (a) A small box measuring about $2 \times 2 \times 1/2$ inches is placed under the skin just below the clavicle (collar bone), and is attached to wires (called leads) introduced into the heart which are responsible for sensing (and recording) the heart rhythm, and ultimately delivering a defibrillation shock when necessary, which restores normal electrical activity. Courtesy of Medtronic Inc. (b, c, d) Examples of ICD generators. Courtesy of Medtronic Inc., St. Jude Medical, Inc. and Boston Scientific.

Patients must also be aware of the possible complications associated with ICDs such as false-shocks due to fast but benign heart rates. Furthermore, there is a small chance of infection, and problems with the leads, including breakage, are not uncommon and may require removal. There have recently been industry-based recalls of defective leads and generators that have affected HCM patients. Although frustrating and unsettling, these

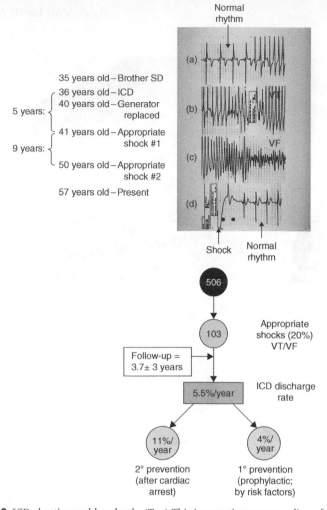

Figure 30 ICD aborting sudden death. (Top) This is a continuous recording of an electrocardiogram obtained from the recording system of the ICD at the time of a life-saving event in a 36-year-old man with HCM. This patient, who had not previously experienced symptoms, received his ICD prophylactically because of high-risk status (extreme wall thickening and sudden HCM death in his younger brother). For almost 5 years, nothing adverse occurred. (a) Then, early one morning while he was asleep at 1 a.m., normal heart rhythm converted suddenly to a life-threatening rhythm disturbance known as ventricular tachycardia (VT). (b) VT continued and this was sensed by the device (as noted by the box). (c) While the device was charging (for 8 seconds), the situation deteriorated, with VT converting to a particularly serious rhythm known as ventricular fibrillation (VF) in which the ventricles (two lower chambers) fibrillate and do not contract effectively to sustain a measurable blood pressure. (d) The ICD automatically delivered a shock, which immediately converted the patient to a normal heart rhythm. Nine years later, an identical event occurred during sleep. This man is now 56, asymptomatic, and alive because of the ICD. (Bottom) Data from the large "ICD in HCM" registry showing that 20% of high-risk patients have an appropriate intervention from their ICD to abort life-threatening arrhythmias over an average of about 3.5 years following implant. Secondary prevention refers to an implant following a cardiac arrest. Primary prevention refers to patients receiving ICDs prophylactically based only on risk factors. Notably, such patients are usually without symptoms of shortness of breath.

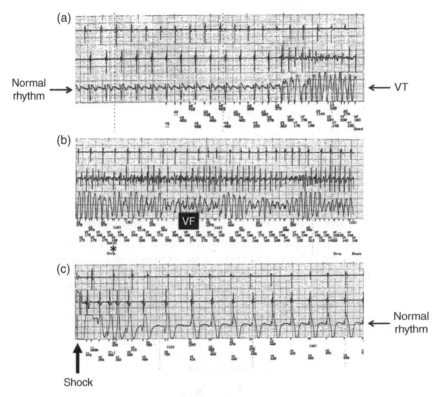

Figure 31 Prevention of sudden death. Recording downloaded from the ICD of a 16-year-old patient who received his device prophylactically because of risk factors for sudden death. (a) The normal rhythm spontaneously, abruptly, and unpredictably converts to a rapid serious rhythm known as ventricular tachycardia (VT). (b) That rhythm deteriorates further to a lethal one, known as ventricular fibrillation (VF). (c) The fully charged ICD, having correctly sensed the situation, delivers a shock (arrow), which "defibrillates" the heart and immediately restores normal rhythm

developments should not discourage HCM patients from decisions for potentially life-saving ICD treatment.

As the risk period in HCM is characteristically very long (theoretically 20–50 years in some patients), the ICD is likely to be a lifelong treatment, thereby creating the crucial necessity for careful and consistent mainte-nance and interrogation of the device (usually 3–4 times per year), as well as regular battery replacement (currently at about 5-year intervals). We have knowledge of several HCM patients in whom the ICD discharged appropriately for the first time as long as almost 10 years after it was first implanted, as well as other patients who have survived for 25 or more

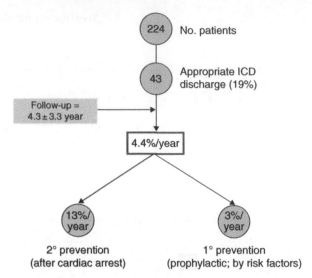

Figure 32 Prevention of sudden death in children. Results of defibrillator study in high-risk children and adolescents <20 years of age with implants. Data are very similar to those for populations comprised largely of adults with HCM. About 20% of the children had appropriate interventions to terminate life-threatening arrhythmias (about 3%/year) when the ICD was implanted prophylactically (primary prevention). Secondary prevention means patients received ICDs after surviving a cardiac arrest. ICD, implantable cardioverter defibrillator.

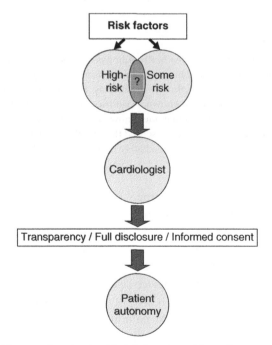

Figure 33 Decision tree for ICDs in HCM. When the evidence for a prophylactic ICD is ambiguous (in a "gray zone"), it is best for your cardiologist to practice transparency and full disclosure with the final decision made by a fully informed patient (inconjunction with the cardiologist).

years after cardiac arrest (without recurrence or ICD shock). In other patients, the ICD discharges earlier (sometimes within the first 6 months). These observations emphasize the unpredictable timing of these potentially lethal events and also the distinct possibility that they may occur only occasionally over a lifetime.

In the future, we expect that ICDs will be offered as life-saving protection to many HCM patients because of high-risk status, prophylactically, before major problems arise. However, it is important to note that ICD is not a treatment for all HCM patients – only for those who are judged by their cardiologist to be at unacceptably increased risk. In high-risk patients, there is no longer a role for antiarrhythmic drugs (such as amiodarone) as a primary alternative to ICD. These medications have not been shown to abolish the risk for sudden death in absolute terms, but are likely to create important side effects over the expected long risk period for young HCM patients. Alternatively, your electrophysiologist may elect to use amiodarone (or other cardioactive drugs, such as beta-blockers) after defibrillator implantation to decrease the likelihood of appropriate or inappropriate shocks during exercise.

- Patients with one or more risk factors can be considered for ICD.
- Only a minority of patients with HCM will need an ICD.
- Those with ICDs can live very active lives.
- ICDs are compatible with most activities and occupations.

Special considerations for implantable defibrillators

Patients and their families may have numerous questions about the ICD and how it might change their lives, particularly since it is likely to represent a chronic treatment (Table 4). Many of these questions should be answered by the electrophysiologist responsible for your device, since these issues may differ on a case-by-case basis, and should be tailored to your own clinical situation and activity level. Regarding questions about the potential interaction between the ICDs and electromagnetic fields in

Table 4 What to expect from an implantable cardioverter defibrillator (ICD).

- Normally, the device is implanted in your upper chest, slightly below your collarbone; you will have a scar about 2 inches long. The leads are introduced through a vein.
- The first implant creates more discomfort than a replacement because a "pocket" is created.
- Bring a button-down shirt to leave the hospital in, as you will not be able to lift your arm over your head for a few days to 2 weeks.
- The use of modern conscious sedation minimizes any discomfort to the patient and eliminates the need for general anesthesia.
- Your leads need time to set within your heart, so you will not be able to lift anything over 10 pounds for a few weeks. You should be able to drive in 1–2 weeks. Talk to your electrophysiologist about specific time frames for returning to work, driving, and lifting, as the time may vary depending on your personal situation.
- Watch for signs of infection when you get home from the hospital; should you start to run a fever, notify your doctor at once.
- If your device delivers a shock, and you are feeling satisfactory afterwards, let your doctor or nurse know. You can wait until normal business hours to contact them. However, if you receive multiple shocks, are feeling ill afterwards, or you still perceive your heart is racing or beating too slowly, you should call 911 (emergency).
- Let someone at work know about your device. In the event that your ICD shocks you while at work, make sure a coworker can help you get the care you may need.
- If a child, teen, or young adult is having a device implanted, you may want to talk to his or her friends and their parents to explain the ICD. Young people spend a great deal of time with friends, and it is important that they know what to do in the event of a shock and also that life with an ICD is not so unusual.
- You must have your ICD checked every few months, the average is 3–4 months, but this varies somewhat from center to center.
- ICDs are hand-made items, and thus subject to imperfection. This is rare, but it can occur. In the event your device is "recalled," do not panic. This does not necessarily mean that your ICD must be removed and replaced. For example, it may mean that programming has to be changed or that the device needs to be assessed for a specific (and correctable) problem.
- If your ICD "beeps," you should notify your electrophysiologist immediately.

the environment, it is important to first understand the nature of an electromagnetic field, which is an invisible line of force resulting from electricity use, such as devices plugged into an outlet or operated by a battery.

Most of the equipment and appliances patients come into contact with on a daily basis will not affect an ICD. However, it is generally a good idea for patients to keep their distance from devices that generate large amounts of electromagnetic interference such as industrial welding instruments, antitheft systems frequently found in stores, and large electrical generators (such as power plants), diathermy, electrocautery, as well as MRI devices. Nevertheless, ICD recipients should be able to safely operate most household appliances, tools, and machines that are properly grounded and in good repair. Some examples that do *not* cause interference include

- Microwave ovens
- Metal detectors
- Televisions, AM/FM radios, videocassette recorders (VCRs)
- Tabletop appliances such as electric toasters, blenders, knives, and can-openers
- Handheld items such as shavers and hair-dryers
- Electric blankets and heating pads
- Major appliances including washers, dryers, and electric stoves
- Personal computers, photocopiers, and electric typewriters
- Light industrial equipment such as drills and table saws (*not* including battery-powered tools)
- Dental drills

Defibrillators are sensitive to particularly strong electrical or magnetic fields, which have the potential to deactivate some devices, although this occurs only on very rare occasions. In some cases, an ICD device may emit a sound if it is too close to a magnet. If this happens, it is important to move away from the object and location immediately. The potential sources of strong electrical and magnetic fields in the following list should be kept at least 12 inches (30 cm) away from an ICD pulse generator:

- Stereo speakers from large systems, transistor radios, "boom boxes," or similar instruments
- Possibly some digital cell phones
- Engines with alternators emitting magnetic fields
- Strong magnets
- Magnetic wands used by airport security, and in other circumstances
- Battery-powered cordless power tools such as screwdrivers and drills

Airport security alarm systems (both the portals through which a person walks or the handheld wand) employ magnetic fields for the purpose of detecting metal. The security portals, or archway, will not harm the device, but it is prudent to walk through at a normal pace and not linger near them. However, the handheld wand used by airport security personnel could deactivate some ICD devices if held directly over the pulse generator for a relatively short period of time. For this reason, ICD identification and security cards should be shown to airport security personnel and patients are encouraged to request an alternative hand search. If security personnel insist on using the wand, the procedure should be performed quickly, and the wand should not linger over the device. New scanning technology offers an alternative to metal detectors, and according to the US Food and

Drug Administration (FDA), the new device known as a backscatter X-ray machine meets the standard of a "general-use" X-ray machine, meaning that a person would have to have 1000 scans a year before approaching the maximum allowable radiation dose for the general public. These devices have no interaction with ICDs or pacemakers.

Patients with ICDs are also discouraged (or restricted) from certain occupations, such as truck, bus, or limousine driver, fireman, police officer, or commercial airline pilot. However, there are a number of police officers and firefighters still working on active duty with ICDs in place after a case-by-case review.

The reliability of implantable devices has come under scrutiny recently and it is important to understand the facts behind this situation. ICDs are highly effective, but these are man-made devices, and flaws will inevitably be identified and corrective action taken. A situation that attracted high public visibility in 2005 involved a number of recalled defibrillators from one manufacturer (Guidant, now Boston Scientific). This circumstance was, in many ways, unique and particularly unfortunate. In this instance, the manufacturer did not disclose to physicians, patients, and the FDA critical information regarding defective defibrillators that could short-circuit, fail, and result in death (initially occurring to a 21-year-old college student with HCM). Subsequently, there have been recalls of leads made by other companies, specifically the Sprint Fidelis (Medtronic) and Riata (St. Jude).

Now, the device manufacturers are working toward better ways to communicate such problems to physicians and patients. ICDs have saved thousands of lives and will save thousands more. Patients with HCM should not allow the events of 2005 to contaminate their trust in ICDs and those cardiologists who recommend and promote this life-saving therapy. To keep up to date on the reliability of your device, we recommend you maintain contact with the manufacturer of your device via their Internet sites or by telephone, and request the most recent information on your device at least once or twice a year. You can also talk to your electrophysiologist at the time of the ICD/pacemaker interrogation to inquire about reliability statistics.

Surgery

Surgery (the **ventricular septal myectomy** operation) is reserved for those patients with marked outflow obstruction who have severe symptoms uncontrolled by treatment with medications (Figure 34, Figure 35,

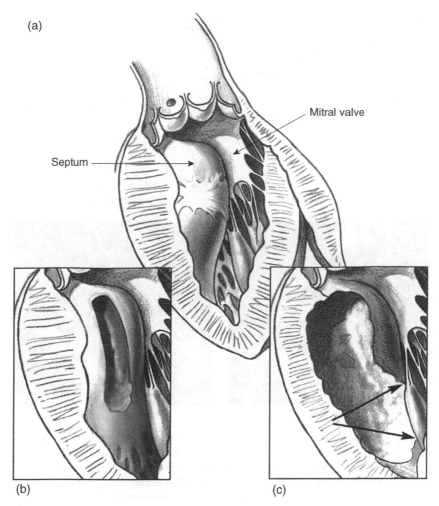

(a)

Mitral valve

Septum

(b)   (c)

Figure 34 Diagram showing two operative approaches for performing septal myectomy in obstructive HCM. (a) Typical outflow tract structure with thickening of the
upper septum and obstruction due to systolic anterior motion of the mitral valve.
(b) A standard rectangular myectomy is created from below the aortic valve to a point
just beyond the point of obstruction, allowing for relief of the outflow gradient.
(c) A much more substantial myectomy is performed by combining the standard
operation with an extended muscle resection deeper into the septum. The portion
of the myectomy toward the bottom of the left ventricle is much wider (arrows).

and Figure 36). The purpose of myectomy is to relieve symptoms of
shortness of breath, and it is an effective and time-proven therapy in this
regard over 40 years. Such symptoms are, in fact, reversible by myectomy.
Surgery is not performed for the purpose of reducing sudden death risk,
although there is some evidence that risk may be reduced by operation.

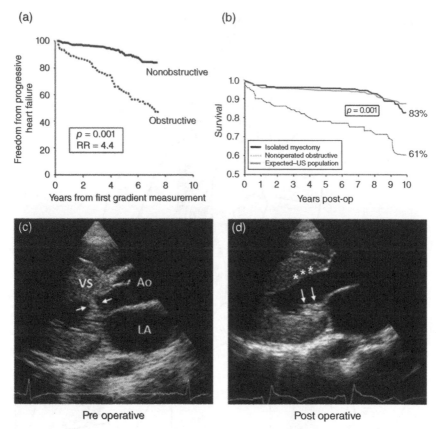

Figure 35 Obstruction in HCM. (a) Obstruction promotes progressive heart failure in many patients, in comparison to patients without obstruction. (b) Survival of HCM patients (considering all causes of mortality) many years after myectomy, compared to survival in the general US population. There is no difference between the two curves and therefore myectomy can be considered a treatment that restores a patient's otherwise expected longevity. Also shown with much less favorable survival for comparison are HCM patients without obstruction, who for some reason did not have myectomy. (c, d) Echocardiograms before and after myectomy. In (c), before operation, systolic anterior motion (SAM) of the mitral valve makes contact with the septum (arrows), causing obstruction; in (d), muscle has been removed from the septum (***), and as a result this valve motion has been obliterated (arrows), and obstruction relieved.

However surgery should not be thought of as a "cure" for HCM because it does not eliminate the entire disease process.

The usual level of obstruction necessary to recommend surgery is a gradient of at least 50 mmHg either at rest or with exercise. With septal myectomy, the operating surgeon removes a small portion of the thickened

Septal scarring

Post ablation   Post myectomy

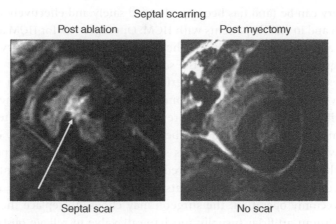

Septal scar   No scar

Figure 36 Distinctive difference between surgical myectomy and alcohol ablation. (Left) Scarring of ventricular septum, which results from the introduction of 95% alcohol. (Right) Myectomy does not produce a scar.

muscle (only 5–10 g in weight) from the upper portion of the ventricular septum, thereby widening the left ventricular cavity in that region, making it unlikely that the mitral valve will contact the septum in systole, thereby relieving the obstruction. Surgeons now more frequently perform what is known as "extended" myectomy, which removes tissue deeper into the ventricle with restructuring of the papillary muscles (Figure 34). Relief of obstruction by myectomy is virtually always permanent.

Surgery for HCM should be performed only by surgeons familiar and experienced with this particular operation (usually at referral centers). HCM surgical candidates should keep this important point in mind when choosing a surgeon. The American College of Cardiology (ACC)/AHA guidelines recommend that surgery be performed at medical centers (and by surgeons) with myectomy experience (defined as a volume of 20 or more operations annually). This has created a situation where HCM patients requiring surgery have frequently traveled outside of their home communities for treatment. In experienced centers, operative mortality is now remarkably low (1% or less), with most patients reporting long-lasting and significant improvement or abolition of symptoms. Moreover, by following large numbers of patients for many years after myectomy, we now understand that longevity after this surgery is similar to that for the general population, and also better than for patients with obstruction who do not undergo myectomy.

Surgery can be (and has been) performed safely and effectively in both children and in elderly patients with HCM. Operative risk for HCM appears to increase some when additional heart surgery (such as coronary artery bypass grafting) is performed at the same time.

If the myectomy operation is performed properly, obstruction will be virtually obliterated under resting conditions and will not return. Therefore, heart failure due to obstruction is a reversible condition when treated with myectomy. Myectomy should only be performed by surgeons fully experienced with this operation. Patients should keep this important point in mind when they are being considered as a candidate for surgical intervention. Occasionally, in selected patients under special circumstances, instead of a myectomy operation, the surgeon may choose to replace the mitral valve with an artificial (usually mechanical) valve to relieve obstruction and symptoms. As surgical complications related to myectomy have decreased dramatically, some have asked why this operation is not performed in less symptomatic (or even asymptomatic) patients. However, as any cardiac surgery, myectomy (although now performed with a high degree of safety in the most experienced centers) is not without some risk. Moreover, it should be underscored that while myectomy removes obstruction, normalizes pressure within the left ventricle, relieves symptoms, reverses heart failure, and extends survival, it is nevertheless not a disease cure; and after surgery patients continue to have HCM with other complications (such as atrial fibrillation) possible.

Of course, some patients who meet the clinical criteria for surgery are not, in fact, optimal candidates for operation – either because of other complicating noncardiac diseases, geographic inaccessibility to an experienced surgeon, particularly advanced age, or fear or lack of motivation for surgery.

Alcohol septal ablation (nonsurgical myectomy)

More recently, an alternative procedure for symptomatic patients with outflow obstruction has been devised to reduce the thickening of the upper septum (and thereby relieve outflow obstruction), without the need for open-heart surgery. Indeed, alcohol septal ablation appears to reduce obstruction and symptoms almost to the same degree as surgery.

This technique involves injecting a small amount of absolute alcohol (about 2 ml) into a minor (small) branch of the left coronary artery that supplies the top portion of the ventricular septum, thus destroying heart cells and ultimately thinning that portion of the wall – and in effect, intentionally producing a myocardial infarction and healed scar (i.e., a "heart attack"). The cavity of the left ventricle is thereby widened, permitting easier and more effective emptying of blood into the aorta – similar to the effects of myectomy. This technique is performed as part of a cardiac catheterization under local anesthesia. Although in a relatively early stage of development (compared to surgery), alcohol ablation represents a useful addition to the management options available to some selected HCM patients with severe drug-refractory HCM symptoms.

However, there are some important issues concerning alcohol ablation worth considering. The overall procedural mortality for the ablation procedure is no less and may exceed that for myectomy (when surgery is performed in experienced centers). At present, the extent to which alcohol septal ablation should be performed in HCM patients remains a somewhat controversial and largely unresolved issue. Some interventional cardiologists advocate it with great enthusiasm, while other cardiologists (including virtually all HCM experts) suggest much more restraint; indeed, there is concern that ablations are being performed excessively by cardiologists new to this technique, and possibly in some patients with fewer symptoms than usually required for the traditional surgical candidate. Caution is advised in making decisions regarding surgery versus ablation.

Notably, all major cardiovascular societies have issued recommendations and guidelines for myectomy versus alcohol ablation – ACC, AHA, and European Society of Cardiology – and each regard myectomy as the preferred ("gold standard") and the primary strategy for most obstructive HCM patients with drug-refractory, severe symptoms and disability.

Alcohol septal ablation is an acceptable treatment option largely in selected HCM patients. These include patients who are of particularly advanced age with associated medical conditions that increase the risk of surgery, lack of sufficient motivation, or have a strong preference against undergoing heart surgery, and importantly have suitable cardiac anatomy for the procedure. Therefore, alcohol ablation is intended to be a potential *alternative to surgery*.

Alcohol ablation leaves patients with a heart scar that can predispose to important arrhythmias (in contrast to surgical myectomy, which leaves no such scar). For these reasons, septal ablation is not recommended for young or even most middle-aged adult patients (and certainly not children). HCM referral institutions perform alcohol septal ablation only in operative candidates who otherwise are not optimal subjects for myectomy. Nevertheless, ablation is a potentially useful addition to the available treatment strategies for selected patients with obstruction and severe symptoms. Also, the anatomy of the left ventricle and mitral valve apparatus, precise location of the obstruction within the chamber, and the size and distribution of the coronary arteries used in the ablation procedure may vary considerably among patients, making some individuals less optimal candidates for alcohol ablation but more likely to benefit from surgery.

- Myectomy is the "gold standard" and preferred treatment for the relief of obstruction in most HCM patients.
- Myectomy now has low operative mortality rate in experienced centers.
- For those patients with suitable anatomy who are of advanced age, alcohol septal ablation can be an alternative to myectomy.
- Both procedures should be performed at centers with high volume (minimum 20 cases per year).
- The goal of septal reduction is to relieve symptoms caused by obstruction – it is not a cure for HCM.
- *Heart failure due to obstruction is reversible in HCM.*

Pacemakers

Pacemakers are used in HCM for several reasons. Occasionally, when the normal electrical signal fails to traverse the ventricles, either because of sinus node failure or heart block, implanting a pacemaker is appropriate and necessary. This involves placing a small box containing a battery in the chest under the skin and passing fine wires through the veins to the heart in order to deliver the necessary signals so that the heart is automatically paced.

In the 1990s, many severely symptomatic patients with HCM and obstruction received dual-chamber pacemakers for the purpose of relieving symptoms and outflow obstruction, as a treatment alternative to the septal myectomy operation. However, much of the symptom improvement perceived by most patients was ultimately shown to be a **placebo effect** rather than a real change in the disease state, and was associated with only modest reduction in the gradient. It is essential to keep in mind that the most important issue in the treatment of any patient with HCM is whether an intervention (e.g., pacing) improves symptoms and quality of life, and not necessarily its precise effect on the degree of obstruction.

In a small number of patients who have progressed to the "end stage" (discussed elsewhere in this book), biventricular pacing has been used to help the heart maintain synchrony and to increase ejection fraction. The use of biventricular pacing requires more research to know whether it has applications to HCM.

- Pacing has a limited role in HCM for reducing symptoms or gradient.
- Pacing features in ICDs provide "backup pacing" and should not be confused with a stand-alone pacemaker.

Heart transplantation and end-stage HCM

For a very small minority of HCM patients (about 2–3%), heart transplantation may be recommended when there is severe, progressive disability and uncontrolled symptoms of shortness of breath with exertion usually associated with impaired heart contraction. This part of HCM is often unfortunately labeled as the "end stage" (or sometimes the "dilated" or "burned-out" phase) and is the most common indication for heart transplantation within the disease spectrum of HCM. The only predictor of "end stage" is a family history of the end stage. The "end stage" represents an instance in the natural history of HCM characterized by a dramatic change in the structure and function of the left ventricle. This occurs by a widespread gradual but irreversible scarring process leading to thinning of the left ventricular wall and enlargement of the heart chambers, impaired pumping capacity, and unfavorable clinical course. Therefore, given our knowledge of the "end-stage" model, the goal of "curing" HCM by therapeutically reducing wall thickness does not appear to be a realistic aspiration in this disease.

Fortunately, the "end stage" is uncommon. Evolution to this phase of the disease occurs spontaneously and without a triggering clinical event. This process results in a form of heart failure more reminiscent of other diseases with greatly enlarged chambers (such as the dilated form of cardiomyopathy). As a result, the medical treatment for the end stage, prior to heart transplantation, will differ considerably from that typically employed in HCM, including administration of beta-blockers (metoprolol, carvedilol), ACE inhibitors (lisinopril, ramipril), angiotensin-receptor blockers (losartan, valsartan, and others), and diuretics. Cardiologists may also choose to prescribe digoxin or spironolactone, and start an anticoagulant treatment. Occasionally, patients with very "stiff" ventricles may require heart transplant even though contraction (in systole) remains normal.

When end stage is identified, patients are advised to contact a transplantation program in their state of residence and obtain their perspective on the requirements of being "listed" for heart transplant. The primary reason for this advice is that sometimes, after being stable for many years, patient's symptoms in the end-stage phase can progress rapidly and unpredictably. The process of evaluation for heart transplantation can take several months, and can be a daunting task for severely symptomatic and disabled patients. After transplantation, patients have a restored quality of life and in almost all cases can go back to their daily routine and jobs – and feel as good as they did before the end-stage process started. However, this "new lease of life" comes at the price of taking immunosuppressive drugs to prevent rejection of the transplanted heart, and compliance with post-transplantation medical appointments. Survival after transplants with HCM is as good as or better than with other diseases: 1-, 5-, and 10-year overall survival of 85, 75, and 61%, respectively, compared to non-HCM transplant patients (82, 70, 49%, respectively). Some HCM patients have survived more than 20 years with a new heart.

It is evident from this discussion that HCM is a particularly heterogeneous disease, and certainly that concept applies directly to the selection of treatment options. The disease and treatment spectrum of HCM are summarized in Figure 28, Figure 37, and Figure 38.

- Patients with HCM can live long and relatively normal lives, even aspiring to normal longevity.
- HCM is now a contemporary treatable disease and patients who develop complications of HCM can be treated with medications or other effective interventions.
- HCM is not a uniformly unfavorable disease but rather a contemporary and treatable condition.
- Lack of symptoms does not mean absence of risk.
- Many patients do not require major treatment interventions. Even patients without symptoms require regular surveillance.

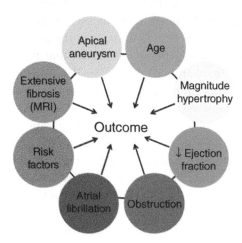

Figure 37 What counts in HCM? HCM is a complex disease, in which several features can potentially influence the clinical course of patients.

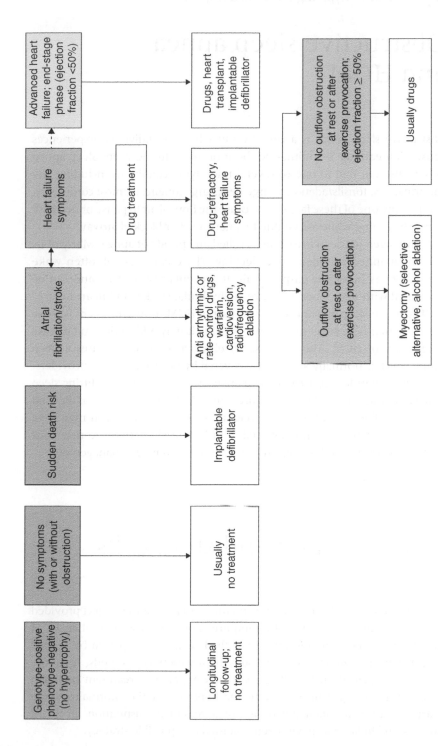

Figure 38 Summary of treatment strategies for the very broad and diverse HCM disease spectrum.

Obstructive sleep apnea and HCM

Obstructive sleep apnea is a condition in which an individual experiences pauses in breathing 5–30 times per hour or more during sleep. Sleep apnea may be present due to one of several underlying conditions including jaw abnormalities, tonsils/adenoids, large neck, large tongue, or, most commonly, obesity. Any one of these factors can cause the flow of air to pause or decrease during breathing while asleep due to a narrowed or blocked airway.

A prolonged pause in breathing is called an episode of apnea. Many of us have brief apnea episodes while sleeping. These episodes will often wake the sleeper as he or she gasps for air. It prevents restful sleep and can be associated with high blood pressure, arrhythmia, stroke, and heart failure.

Obstructive sleep apnea is not *per se* part of HCM. However, there is some literature that now suggests in some patients it may add to risk and disease progression of HCM. The diagnosis of obstructive apnea requires a sleep study, which is normally an expense covered by health insurance providers.

The treatment for obstructive sleep apnea is a breathing mask during sleep called a continuous positive airway pressure (*CPAP*) device, as well as diet and exercise modification to promote weight loss. If you suspect you may have sleep apnea or have been diagnosed with it, you should ensure that your cardiologist knows of this diagnosis to aid in your complete management.

Gene therapy and stem cells

Given the visibility of gene therapy and the human genome project provided by the news media, patients often inquire about the possibility of an HCM cure through gene therapy (in which "bad" genes are replaced by "good" genes) delivered directly into the body by a variety of methods. It is very unlikely that gene therapy will be a workable or practical treatment approach for HCM. Reducing wall-thickening and hypertrophy (i.e., normalizing the heart structure) by such means is not a reasonable aspiration for HCM patients and in fact has never been regarded as a possible strategy.

Conceptually, gene therapy will be a very difficult process in a disease genetically transmitted as a dominant trait (such as HCM). Standard models for which this treatment has been proposed are other types of genetic diseases with **recessive transmission**. Also, gene therapy does not seem applicable to HCM since the notion of introducing enough "good genes" to make all the cells normal is regarded by molecular scientists as particularly daunting. Furthermore, such a treatment would not be without risk to patients, raising ethical issues as to which patients could (or should) be treated in this way. Keep in mind that many (if not most) HCM patients experience a relatively benign course, and can achieve normal life expectancy, without heroic interventions. Therefore, in purely theoretical terms, gene therapy (even if possible) would necessarily have very limited application and be confined to particularly high-risk HCM patients and families, and specifically very young patients in whom hypertrophy is not fully established. It is evident that (even if technically feasible) the selection of HCM patients for gene therapy could be as complex as the treatment itself.

Therapy for cardiovascular and other diseases with stem cells is currently an area of intense interest and study, and also media focus. However, stem cell therapy would not appear to be applicable to HCM since adding heart cells to a disease state in which the heart is already excessively thickened would not make sense or be advisable.

Automated external defibrillators (AEDs)

Early defibrillation, especially when delivered within 3–5 minutes of a collapse from SCA provides the best chance for survival. AEDs can be used by just about anyone with minimal training; in fact, children in elementary school have been trained and showed ample understanding to use the device appropriately. The AED is a potentially life-saving device, now widely available for use in community settings or in private homes. The AED is designed to automatically analyze the electrical activity of the heart and determine whether a "shockable" rhythm is present. With voice prompts, the AED is programmed to guide rescuers (even the untrained) through the resuscitation process and issue instructions regarding when to initiate a shock.

Patients often ask: "Should I have an AED in my home rather than having an ICD implanted?" The answer is simply no; an AED is not as dependable as an ICD and you must have a person with you who witnesses the event and employs the device. It is simply not practical to take an AED with you everywhere you go and it offers no protection during sleep.

Having an AED in the home is not a "bad" idea for those with HCM and no risk factors, especially if you are in a rural area with slow Emergency Medical Services (EMS) response times. You may wish to speak to your cardiologist about ordering an AED for the home. Some insurance providers will cover the cost of an AED as a durable medical product. Prior to bringing an AED into the home, it is a good idea to discuss this as a family and ensure that everyone understands the reason and that all family members are comfortable enough to use the device if it is needed. Many who work with this technology liken it to having a fire extinguisher in the home.

The HCMA and others have long advocated for the placement of AEDs in schools, community centers, recreation fields, places of employment, and fitness centers. Some states (New York, Pennsylvania, Illinois, and New Jersey to name a few) have laws requiring them in schools while states like Connecticut have language-encouraging AEDs in schools but are not mandating them. There is no legislation mandating AEDs in most states. New Jersey requires AEDs in fitness centers and the Federal Government requires them in all federal buildings. AEDs are safe to be used by bystanders, but many devices have a warning label indicating that they are to be used only by trained personnel (there is no federal regulation mandating this language). This caution label is controversial.

HCM as a chronic disease: Is a cure available?

HCM is just one of many chronic diseases, such as diabetes, coronary artery disease, or inflammatory bowel disease. In this sense, chronic means not completely reversible, but nevertheless does *not* mean untreatable. HCM is, in fact, a contemporary treatable disease. Although HCM cannot be eradicated or cured, it is a disease that can be controlled allowing extended longevity with good quality of life. *All complications of HCM have treatments which have proven effective for most patients.*

However, adjustment to the diagnosis of any chronic disease takes *time.* There is no satisfactory alternative to time. A diagnosis such as HCM is shocking, and attacks any person's sense of vulnerability. The new diagnosis of HCM makes a patient suddenly vulnerable, no matter how benign the particular disease expression appears to be. When first diagnosed, the idea of HCM is daunting, but as time passes it becomes a part of daily living, requiring attention to taking medications and ensuring proper hydration, as well as a healthy diet and exercise program. Periodically, it may take more energy and time, for example, with ICD checks and cardiology visits.

Patients often ask whether there is a known cure for HCM. If "cure" means complete and absolute elimination of the entire disease process and all of its consequences, then HCM is not curable, and likely will not be so in our lifetime. However, in this regard, it is also very important to emphasize that the disease process can be controlled in most patients and HCM is compatible with normal longevity, not uncommonly with little or no disability and without the need for major treatment interventions. The more serious disease complications can often be managed and controlled with drugs, surgery, or implantable devices.

Therefore, HCM does not necessarily shorten life or impact substantially the quality of life. For example, in patients judged to be at high risk for sudden death, an ICD will likely be protective from such an event. For that individual patient, there may be no other risks related to HCM and therefore the ICD could possibly be regarded as a "cure," that is, allowing that patient to achieve normal or near-normal longevity. It will, however, take many years of observations in large patient populations to confirm this hypothesis.

Nevertheless, many patients with HCM continue to live with the fear that their life is destined to be short, based solely on the diagnosis of HCM. This is not correct and very short-sighted. While HCM can be life-threatening, it is treatable. This paradox is often the cause for confusion, frustration, and denial for many patients. Many HCMA members are enjoying long, meaningful, and healthy lives. With the advances in our understanding of HCM, and with early diagnosis and treatment, it is reasonable to expect that life spans will continue to be long, if not longer than in past generations, for those with this complex disease. Furthermore, a life with minimal or no significant medical intervention is not only possible but is in fact common for those with HCM.

Are you newly diagnosed?

If you are newly diagnosed with HCM, there are many emotions and thoughts to deal with and there is no one right or wrong way to process this information. It is very individualistic, but there are a number of specific issues to consider (Table 5). You should expect to encounter emotions similar to that which we face when dealing with a death; this may be in part because those diagnosed with HCM feel as though they have suffered a loss of part of themselves and become vulnerable, that is, the lost perception of what is "normal" and "healthy" with the recognition that they have a chronic and possibly life-threatening condition. For others, it may be a tie

Table 5 Checklist for the newly diagnosed with HCM

---

1 Speak to your cardiologist about his or her experience level with HCM.

2 Ask your cardiologist about his or her feelings on working in partnership with an HCM specialty center to manage your care.

3 Make sure all tests have been performed to ensure thorough risk stratification:
  (a) Echocardiogram
  (b) Electrocardiogram
  (c) Holter monitor
  (d) Stress test/stress echo
  (e) Cardiac MRI (with contrast)

4 Discuss with your doctor your treatment options:
  (a) If medications are prescribed, make sure you are clear on the dosage, timing, and side effects you may encounter, and when to talk to your cardiologist.
  (b) If an ICD or pacemaker is recommended, make sure you consult with an electrophysiologist prior to implantation.
  (c) If surgery is recommended, make sure you ask how many procedures have been performed at the center and how often they are down. HCMA highly recommends only centers which regularly perform myectomies, and have many years of experience in this operation.
  (d) If you have been recommended for alcohol septal ablation (also known as PTSMA or TASHO, we suggest a complete evaluation by an HCM specialty center and careful adherence to the American College of Cardiology (ACC)/European Society of Cardiology (ESC) Consensus Document guidelines on the treatment of HCM.

5 Discuss your employment situation with your cardiologist and make sure you can safely perform the duties required. If you cannot perform at work, ask your physician to write a letter to your Human Resources Department with a request for an Americans with Disabilities Act Accommodation.

6 Notify family members that they should have screening for HCM. The screening should include an ECG, echocardiogram, consultation with a cardiologist, and a plan for future screening on an age-appropriate basis.

---

to their family history which may have included the death or disability of a relative. The stages you may encounter include the following.

1 *Shock and denial*

You may react to learning of the diagnosis with numbed disbelief. You may deny the reality of the diagnosis at some level, in order to avoid the pain. Shock provides emotional protection from being overwhelmed. This may last for weeks.

2 *Pain and guilt*

As the shock wears off, it may be replaced with the suffering of pain and guilt, which is called "genetic guilt" at the HCMA. It is important that you experience the pain fully, and not hide it, avoid it, or escape from it with alcohol, drugs, or deeper denial. Life feels chaotic and scary during this phase. Once you have felt the guilt, release it as it has no value and nothing positive can come of it. You may develop an acute awareness of your heart and every little sensation may be exaggerated in your mind. We refer to this as being very "cardiac aware" – in all likelihood, these symptoms may have been present for years; however, your former belief that this was a "normal" state has now been replaced by "abnormal" because you have HCM.

3 *Anger and bargaining*

Frustration gives way to anger, and you may lash out and lay unwarranted blame for the diagnosis on someone else. Try to control this, as permanent damage to your relationships may result. This is a time for release of bottled-up emotion. You may rail against fate, questioning "Why me?" You may also try to bargain in vain with powers that may exist for a way out of your despair: "Please make my heart better and I will do good for the world."

4 *"Depression," reflection, loneliness*

Just when your friends may think you should be getting on with your life, a long period of sad reflection will likely overtake you. This is a normal stage of grief, so do not be "talked out of it" by well-meaning outsiders. Encouragement from others is not helpful to you during this stage of grieving.

During this time, you finally realize the true magnitude of your diagnosis, and it may depress you. You may isolate yourself on purpose, reflect on things you did prior to your diagnosis, and focus on memories of the past. You may sense feelings of emptiness and despair.

5 *The upward turn*

As you start to adjust your life with your diagnosis, you become a little calmer and more organized. Your physical symptoms appear to lessen, and your "depression" begins to lift.

6 *Reconstruction and working through*
As you become more functional, your mind starts working again, and you find yourself seeking realistic solutions to problems posed by life with HCM. You start to work on practical and financial problems and reconstructing yourself and your life with HCM and see that it is not all that different than life before.

7 *Acceptance and hope*
During this, the last of seven stages in this grief model, you learn to accept and deal with the reality of your situation. Acceptance does not necessarily mean instant happiness. Given the pain and turmoil you may have experienced, you can never return to the carefree, untroubled you that existed before your diagnosis. But you will find a way forward. Sometimes you just need to readjust the sails and begin a new journey, and it may be far more exciting and fulfilling than you ever imagined.

Adapting psychologically to HCM

The initial diagnosis of HCM, which often comes as a complete surprise, can actually have a profound psychological impact (Table 5). Furthermore, the effect of chronic illness (such as HCM) on a patient and family is similar to that of other emotional trauma. Chronic diseases produce the feelings of fear, grief, and loss that are essentially unending. HCM (which often affects young people and conveys a risk for sudden cardiac death in some patients) presents patients and their families with a lack of predictability, which itself may make adjustment to life more difficult. There is constant living with the unknown and an acute sense that any personal control over events is lacking. In contrast, in most other instances of loss, as terrible as they are, there is at least a finality that must be accepted; shock and denial give way to acceptance and adaptation.

Imagine the following scenario. Someone says to you: "Carry this beeper. One day it may go off and you must respond immediately and correctly. It will be the most important moment of your life. It could go off next week, next year, or 10 years from now but be ready." This situation can create chronic anxiety and anger in patients, their family, and friends, and thus is essentially what happens with a disease such as HCM. A medical condition can itself become an anxiety state characterized by preoccupation and hyperalertness, and can paralyze the patient's adjustment to daily-life activities. Eventually, depression can result when the constant state of readiness (and often a sense of hopelessness) gradually wears down the patient's reserves. There is often a profound sense of unfairness ("how and why did this happen to me"), but also the realization that life is fragile and imperfect. The trauma created by chronic diseases can also result in reprioritization of life goals and values – which may represent a positive consequence of an otherwise negative situation.

Disruption of the family homeostasis and the roles that members have played for years can be thrown into disarray. There may also be substantial guilt involved in HCM families – that is, for having transmitted the gene and disease to children. This may also relate to the dilemma faced by many patients, of deciding to have children (and take the chance of transmitting the mutant gene).

"Genetic guilt" is a natural emotion on the part of a parent affected by HCM who has a child with HCM. However, if a parent feels "genetic guilt" over the genetic material that made his or her child's abnormal heart, they should also be prepared to take credit for the wonderful genetic contributions made to create that beautiful smile, loving eyes, adorable laugh, or wonderful sense of humor.

Therefore, *genetic counseling* is an important component of treatment for HCM, as it may help to answer difficult and delicate questions for patients. Certainly, in many families, there is not an absolutely correct answer to questions about HCM, as a number of considerations may be involved, including the variable clinical expression of the gene defect within and between families. Most importantly, for the majority of patients with HCM, it is not necessary to live in terror of the possibility of deterioration and premature death, since it is now evident that this disease is often consistent with normal life expectancy.

Chronic diseases such as HCM present a series of dilemmas and a continuum of choices for patients. As a goal, we recommend achieving a psychological state somewhere in between the following extremes:
• From ignoring your symptoms and "toughing it out" to overreacting to your symptoms.
• From keeping your illness secret and risk deception to talking too openly and risking the perception of self-pity.

- From asking for help and risking becoming a burden to holding on to your independence and risking isolation.
- From insisting that your family and friends treat you as normal and denying them the expression and release of their feelings to letting your family and friends protect you and risk becoming overly dependent or childlike.
- From pushing your body to its physical limits and risking self-harm to playing it safe and becoming an invalid.
- From living in terror of degeneration and death and risking immobilization to regarding each day as a special and pristine opportunity.
- From insisting on controlling your life at the risk of frustration to going with the flow and risking passivity.
- From being angry at your circumstances and risking bitterness to focusing only on your blessings and risking self-delusion.

Fortunately, it is characteristic of human beings that a capacity for strength can be drawn from adversity. This can be aided by mutual support between patients and their families and by interaction between patients afflicted by the same disease. This process includes acknowledging what could have been and accepting and adapting to the reality of the given situation, and also finding ways to make your life meaningful despite a chronic illness. It is important that as many family members and friends as possible participate in this renewal. The family that has been traumatized by chronic illness can thereby take collective pride in a newfound strength.

Finally, patients should refrain from seeking miracle solutions and should be cautious and discriminating about accepting seemingly unrealistic, dramatic predictions about disease cures, regardless of the source. Perhaps, it is best to regard most treatment advances in HCM in the context of *controlling* the disease, rather than as *cures* which obliterate the disease.

- HCM is a chronic disease and patients and their families will likely face a period of adjustment to the diagnosis.
- HCM patients may experience "genetic guilt" for transmitting the condition to their children, but this is wasted energy and should be avoided.
- There is no single right way to acclimate to an HCM diagnosis, but support and communication are important.

Family screening

The majority of patients with HCM have at least one other affected relative (i.e., usually a parent, sibling, or child). When an individual is diagnosed with HCM, all close relatives should be advised and afforded the option of screening for the disease with a personal and family history, echocardiogram, MRI, and ECG. It is important to remember that such a family evaluation is potentially important because HCM may be present, even without associated heart symptoms (Table 2).

The standard screening tests for making the clinical diagnosis of HCM are imaging with two-dimensional echocardiogram (and Doppler), more recently supplemented by cardiac MRI and the 12-lead ECG. The purpose of screening with the echocardiogram/MRI is to identify what is known as the **phenotype** or overt expression of HCM – that is, the abnormal thickening of the left ventricular wall. In this regard, it is important to keep in mind an important distinction. While the mutant gene is present from birth, thickening of the left ventricular wall is delayed and almost always develops later (even decades later, in some cases). Sometimes HCM is referred to as a "congenital" heart disease (present from birth), but it is only the genetic abnormality that is present from conception. This, of course, raises the unresolved question of when HCM becomes a "disease" – at birth, when the mutant gene is present; later, when the heart wall thickens; or if and when symptoms occur. This particular nomenclature can be confusing to patients.

Heart wall thickening is most likely to be detected in the adolescent years and usually increases as children progress through puberty with accelerated body growth and maturation (approximately 12–17 years). Indeed, if a thickened wall becomes evident in an HCM family member on the echocardiogram during adolescence – and cannot be explained in any another way – it may be assumed to represent the gene mutation causing HCM. These changes in thickness with growth can be abrupt and striking and therefore the appearance of the heart can be altered substantially during the teenage years – from completely normal (or near-normal) thickness to a very thick left ventricle. HCM experts believe that these changes in hypertrophy, while often alarming in appearance to the family (and even some physicians), nevertheless represent the expected ("normal") pattern for that individual patient with HCM (dictated by the DNA code), reflecting the way the heart reaches its mature structural form in this genetic disease.

Therefore, the rapid growth of the heart, commonly seen in teenagers, does not *per se* represent clinical deterioration or a warning of imminent danger. In addition, the fear of many patients that their heart will continue to thicken throughout life, ultimately resulting in a catastrophic event, is completely unfounded. In fact, in the vast majority of patients, wall thickness does not increase measurably (and may even decrease slightly) with advancing age in the general adult HCM population (after approximately age 21 years).

Usually, if hypertrophy is not present on the echocardiogram by the time full growth and maturation is achieved (about 17–19 years), then it is less likely for it to appear later in life. However, recent research has shown that this rule is not invariable and some family members may not express their hypertrophy for the first time until midlife or beyond. To date, only a very few genetically affected individuals have been known to develop hypertrophy for the first time after age 30 years, and certainly the frequency with which this phenomenon occurs is unknown. Consequently, for a relative in an HCM family who is "echo-negative" by the time adulthood begins (and with a normal ECG), there is a high likelihood (probably 95% or more) of being an unaffected family member. Of course, if a clinically affected family member is successfully genotyped in the laboratory (i.e., the family HCM mutation has been identified by genetic testing), then uncertainty can be removed since it is then relatively easy to determine whether or not other relatives are affected by the same mutation.

But when should echocardiograms/MRIs be performed routinely in children and other relatives within families with HCM? The current recommendations for clinical screening are summarized in Table 2. Screening echocardiograms before the onset of puberty are largely optional since hypertrophy is rarely evident at that time, and recognition of the disease at this age is not usually accompanied by treatment considerations. One exception to this would be children in selected families with multiple occurrences of premature death due to HCM. In such a circumstance, early identification of high-risk individuals would be advantageous by permitting strategies for the prevention of sudden death to be implemented. Imaging early in life is also recommended for young family members who are engaged in intensive competitive athletic training programs, since HCM is the most important cause of sudden death during sports in young people, and disqualification from that lifestyle is expected to reduce risk. In general, we recommend serial echocardiograms (and ECGs) about every

12–18 months, from the onset of puberty (about 12–13 years) throughout adolescence or until the echocardiogram/MRI "converts" from normal to abnormal (i.e., thickens).

Because of the possibility of "late (adult) onset hypertrophy" into midlife or even beyond, it is probably prudent for asymptomatic relatives with normal echocardiograms and ECGs at 18 years to obtain subsequent echocardiograms (and ECGs) at about 5-year intervals to be sure that their hearts have not "converted" to HCM. This is admittedly a troublesome recommendation since "late-onset hypertrophy" is probably very uncommon, and we know that 50% of those family members with such extended screening would, in fact, be truly normal. This recommendation, of course, assumes that there has not been genetic testing that excluded an HCM mutation.

Strangely enough, the standard ECG may show an abnormal pattern in genetically affected children or some adults long before the echocardiogram/MRI changes from normal to abnormal and with evidence of thickening in the left ventricular wall. Therefore, the ECG can be the first clue or evidence of the HCM gene in young family members. On the other hand, completely normal ECGs are not uncommon in HCM, from 5% in a clinically referred population to 25% in family screening.

Patients often ask whether the HCM gene can "skip" a generation, but rather it is expressed so secretly that its representation cannot be seen even by heart imaging. This is called **incomplete penetrance**.

What about having children? Pregnancy and delivery

Even if a child inherits the abnormal HCM gene, the degree to which he or she will be affected by the disease is largely unpredictable. There is no consistently reliable method for predicting how severe HCM might be in an offspring and, in fact, there is considerable variability in this regard, even within the individual families. A mildly affected parent can have a severely affected child, or vice versa. Alternatively, an entire family may have "benign" disease while other (albeit uncommon) families have "malignant" forms of HCM in which several relatives die prematurely or have severe disease and disability. Therefore, genetic counseling decisions to determine whether or not to have children must be an individual choice, based on many considerations, including the particular expressions of HCM in the family.

For the vast majority of women with HCM, pregnancy and vaginal delivery poses no added risk and is well tolerated and safe. However, in the rare situation when a female HCM patient has severe symptoms or important arrhythmias, pregnancy could carry additional risk, and Caesarean section may be considered selectively to achieve some control over the medical circumstances. Obviously, such symptomatic pregnant woman should have a cardiologist and access to specialized high-risk obstetrical care in order to make many important clinical decisions. Maternal death due to HCM as a consequence of childbirth is extraordinarily rare and virtually unreported in recent years.

However, women may find that they develop symptoms for the first time during pregnancy, or that preexisting symptoms are intensified. Issues related to taking cardiac drugs around the time of conception or during pregnancy arise in many cases. Drugs such as beta-blockers, calcium channel blockers (e.g., verapamil) taken by the mother have access to the fetus because they are capable of crossing the placental barrier, and could in theory damage the baby. However, there is little direct evidence that the fetus can in fact be damaged due to the administration of these drugs to the mother. The one exception is Coumadin. It is simply not compatible with pregnancy and will lead to severe birth defects in the child and potential bleeding risk for the mother. Nevertheless, it is best to be cautious, if possible, and avoid all drugs during pregnancy (certainly in the first trimester). For all these reasons, it is prudent for patients with HCM to plan their pregnancy in advance and discuss all pertinent medical issues at an early stage with their cardiologist and obstetrician. It may also be best to avoid epidural anesthesia at delivery (particularly in women with obstruction), as this occasionally causes an excessive fall in blood pressure and therefore could increase obstruction. It is also safe for most women to breast-feed while on most cardiac medications. However, details should be discussed with your physician.

We are, however, living in a world that allows for the use of technology to assist with family planning in a new and potentially beneficial way. The topic of preimplantation genetic diagnosis (PGD) is one that may be offensive to some based on religious or ethical grounds. Conversely, there are

people with severe expressions of HCM, sometimes reaching back generations, who would benefit from the ability to have a child free of HCM. PGD
allows couples with an increased risk for transmitting a severe and potentially lethal genetic disease like HCM to conceive a child who will not
inherit the pathologic mutation. The concept for PGD requires extremely
precise laboratory methods to ensure the best possible outcome. First, the
person affected with HCM must have genetic testing with definitive results
for a disease-causing mutation. Next, the egg and sperm are harvested
from the parents. This is done in the traditional manner of in vitro fertilization (IVF). After fertilization, the embryo is tested to see if it carries the
HCM mutation. This is performed on a single cell (of the 8-cell, 3-day-old
embryo). Only embryos that do not carry the HCM genetic mutation are
implanted and the remainder of the embryos are discarded.

- The choice to have a child (if one parent has HCM) is a personal one and should be
  given substantial thought prior to conception.
- Pregnancy and delivery is safe for the vast majority of HCM patients.

Routine medical care

Patients with HCM should be seen regularly by a cardiologist near their
home even if they are stable and do not develop new complaints. Clinic
visits on an annual basis seem to work out best. Many patients complain
that their cardiologist openly expresses inexperience with HCM. This, of
course, is not an uncommon occurrence because of the relative infrequency of HCM in the general population and in cardiology practice.
Some patients alleviate this frustration by electing to be evaluated and
followed concurrently by an HCM consultant – that is, a cardiologist
with special interest and expertise in HCM. You may contact the HCMA
for names of HCM specialists (Tel: 973 983 7429; Fax: 973 983 7870;
e-mail: support@4hcm.org). Links to HCM specialty centers can be found
on the HCMA website (www.4HCM.org) or by personally contacting the
HCMA office.

Generally, if HCM patients are stable and new issues do not arise, medical visits no more frequent than at 1-year intervals (with history and

physical examination, echocardiogram, 12-lead ECG, and ambulatory Holter ECG and probably MRI) is customary practice, and an opportunity to reassess risk factors and adjust medications, if necessary. Of course, for those patients who are symptomatic and require treatment, more frequent follow-up may be required with a cardiologist as well as with another sub-specialist such as an electrophysiologist (e.g., if a defibrillator is implanted). Emergency room communication about HCM may be difficult. Therefore, a medic alert bracelet, emergency information card, or Medic Alert USB (available from HCMA) may be of assistance in such rare situations.

Diet

Sensible eating habits are encouraged to maintain body weight within the normal range for height and age. If an individual is overweight, this places unnecessary strain on the HCM heart as would be the case for any cardiac condition. Attention should also be paid to lipid (i.e., cholesterol) levels, as would be advised for any patient. However, we wish to emphasize that cholesterol is a risk factor for coronary artery disease, and not specifically for HCM. No special diet or vitamin supplementation is required for HCM. Of note, a rapid increase in weight is likely to be due to fluid retention and requires consultation with your physician. Excessive salt intake should be avoided, but unless heart failure is in an advanced stage, low-salt diets are not usually advised. Under ideal conditions, the minimum sodium requirement is about 1500 mg each day. This is less than 1 teaspoon of table salt. The maximum recommendation level of sodium intake is 2300 mg per day for the average person.

Exercise

It is important to have a clear understanding of the difference between participation in "competitive sports" and a healthy exercise regimen. Most experts believe individuals with a confirmed diagnosis of HCM should not participate in most organized, competitive sports or other intense physical activities, as discussed in the section on "Special consideration: athletes and sports activities." This recommendation is based on the observation that intense physical exertion appears to predispose some susceptible individuals with HCM to arrhythmias and possibly sudden death.

In many families, sports have been traditional or play a very large role in daily life. These activities may have, in fact, become a major focus and important part of the social life of not only the child but the entire family. After a child has received a diagnosis of HCM, it will be difficult for all parties (regardless of age) to understand that they can no longer participate in competitive sports. Indeed, when a diagnosis of HCM is made in a committed athlete, it is perhaps more devastating in many ways than the same diagnosis in a nonathletic child. Such children will require assistance to redirect their time and energy to other activities (that may include certain recreational sports), or in some cases to more acceptable competitive sports such as golf or bowling. Therefore, it is important to encourage the child to maintain existing relationships with friends in sports, but at the same time extend their network to individuals who participate in other activities. At the same time, it will also be difficult for parents, who also have developed social contacts associated with these sporting events, to no longer be able to participate. Some parents can find it just as difficult to deal with this loss as does the child.

For most patients, HCM will not interfere importantly with lifestyle. Patients with HCM and symptoms such as shortness of breath, chest pain, or lightheadedness during activity (even if mild) should not extend themselves into a physical activity zone which has the effect of provoking or accentuating symptoms. Such symptoms can be regarded as warning signs that heart function has been impaired. It is best to consider the axiom: have a good measure of respect for your disease and do not extend yourself beyond a reasonable threshold.

Nevertheless, after these considerations are taken into account, it is a reasonable expectation that most affected individuals with HCM can adopt a normal or near-normal lifestyle, including many recreational physical activities, as long as they are undertaken in *moderation*. HCM patients should seek the advice of their cardiologist with regard to precisely what type of recreational exercise program should be implemented. In addition, AHA recommendations are available to serve as a useful guide to these difficult decisions (Table 5).

Exercise programs for patients with HCM should not be confused with participation in competitive athletics or certain intense recreational sports. HCM patients are not compelled to lead a completely sedentary lifestyle; in fact, this is discouraged. For example, walking and toning with weights (exclusive of free weights), bicycling, or lap swimming are generally acceptable forms of exercise. However, all systematic exercise programs should be initiated with some caution. If the patient with HCM is seeking to join a gym, careful evaluation of activities is cautioned as well as an understanding of the laws in his or her state; for example, in New Jersey, all public gyms are required to have AEDs and thus offer a small level of protection.

Alcohol

Patients with HCM should avoid excessive consumption of alcohol because of its potentially adverse effects on heart muscle and vasculature. In addition, one study has shown outflow obstruction to actually increase after consuming very small amounts of alcohol, probably due to dilation of peripheral blood vessels produced by the drug. On the other hand, modest intake of beer or wine is certainly acceptable. One should maintain adequate hydration (with water) while consuming alcohol.

Sexual activity/erectile dysfunction

It is important to remember that a healthy sex life is crucial to overall well-being. Those with HCM should be able to enjoy a normal and active sex life without concern for risk associated with their disease. Drugs such as beta-blockers have, however, been responsible for reversible impotence.

Viagra® (sildenafil citrate), Levitra® (vardenafil), and Cialis® (tadalafil) are the drugs available for the treatment of erectile dysfunction for which sudden death and other adverse consequences have been associated in a small number of symptomatic patients with coronary artery disease. However, because HCM is a much less common disease, there are no data specifically governing the side effects of these medications specifically in this disease. Nevertheless, there are certain theoretic reasons to avoid these drugs if you have HCM. Since sidenafil, vardenafil, and tadlafil dilate arterial and venous vessels, they could increase obstruction and in this way be adverse to HCM patients. Therefore, patients with HCM should probably avoid Viagra®, Levitra®, and Cialis® as much as possible until more data are available. Careful consultation with your cardiologist is advised before taking any medications in this class.

Flu vaccination

"Flu shots" may be recommended by your doctor to prevent influenza, particularly in very young and elderly individuals. Having HCM does not exclude this treatment, although you should be aware that there are occasional side effects from the vaccine (which also may not provide absolute protection against infection).

Weight management and obesity in HCM

The medical literature extensively describes the adverse cardiovascular effects of obesity. There are an estimated 75 million or more Americans who are more than 30lb over their ideal body weight. New data specifically in HCM show that excess body weight worsens the degree of heart failure and functional limitation. It stands to reason that patients with HCM who have weight-related medical conditions such as diabetes, systemic hypertension, and coronary artery disease face a far greater likelihood of complications, and a less favorable future, when compared to those of average or normal weight.

Patients with HCM face additional challenges when dealing with long-term weight management issues. Many patients cannot exercise regularly and adopt a sedentary lifestyle out of necessity. Certainly the combination of a sedentary existence and chronic disease such as HCM makes weight loss difficult. Furthermore, since obesity can worsen heart-related symptoms, substantial uncertainty may arise regarding whether symptoms are due to HCM directly or at least in part due to the patient's weight gain. It is critical for such patients to work closely with cardiac professionals to create a strategy and practical physical activity program to reduce weight.

Taking small steps to make long-term changes in eating habits and exercise is the way to start. It is important to remember that you will not necessarily see huge changes over short periods of time. Creating a healthy eating plan in coordination with an exercise program will, however, eventually lead to gradual weight loss, which is more likely to result in true weight loss over time.

Finally, the subject of weight loss to an obese patient itself can create stress, depression, and feelings of failure. However, it is important to directly face the issue to improve overall health and start on the road to weight reduction. This will likely be a trial-and-error process until you find the weight loss method that works best for you. However, fad diets, over-the-counter diet pills, and starvation diets are not the way to safely lose meaningful weight and may in fact be dangerous for those with HCM.

Other restrictions

Acute severe loss of blood or bodily fluid, hemorrhage, diarrhea, and vomiting, if excessive, can lead to unfavorable consequences such as increase in obstruction. Seek medical attention should you experience severe diarrhea or vomiting.

Prolonged standing in excessively hot conditions or very hot baths or showers may predispose to fainting or near-fainting.

Anesthesia: special attention is required to avoid a sudden drop in blood pressure. There have been a few reports suggesting an increased risk associated with epidural anesthesia during delivery; this procedure should probably be avoided in HCM patients, particularly in the presence of outflow obstruction.

Prolonged exposure to extreme environmental temperatures (hot or cold) can predispose to unfavorable consequences including arrhythmias. When exercising, HCM patients should avoid such conditions and maintain hydration in high temperatures whether or not engaged in physical activity.

Community screening for HCM

Screening programs that include ECGs or echocardiograms are being conducted outside of the traditional health-care model in various locations including school gymnasiums, recreation centers, and school nurses' offices. These mass screening programs are often staffed by volunteers (with some medical oversight). There are many issues and concerns about quality, privacy, and reproducibility. Some such programs include ECGs which are known to have false positive and false negative rates in the range of 10–20%. Thus, screening large healthy populations of young people with ECGs to exclude complex cardiovascular disease is not very specific. The use of echocardiograms for HCM screening is theoretically more powerful but creates other concerns since most screening echocardiograms are not performed as complete examinations and use protocols that are variable and with inconsistent quality control. One area of significant concern is that many of these programs suggest to the public that the screening process is comprehensive enough to be diagnostic for most relevant diseases, thereby providing a false sense of security to parents and families.

Community outreach

Many families, patients, and health-care professionals seek ways to raise awareness of HCM and identify the great number of "unidentified" patients. The opportunity to be diagnosed and receive care is a meaningful event, and one some patients wish to share with others. There are several initiatives one can take to help others identify their personal risk for heart disease and HCM, as well as prepare for sudden cardiac arrest (SCA) events in schools and at the workplace. The two programs discussed here focus on efforts that engage, educate, and create systems that are sustainable in partnership with health-care professionals.

A first step is to help identify those who would benefit from additional screening for cardiac disease. While health-care professionals will take a history from a patient, if that patient is unaware of precisely what information they should provide, then important signs and symptoms may be overlooked. Therefore, dissemination of the SCA Risk Assessment Tool, particularly for those under 40 years of age is of potential value. This form contains questions which can help to identify those at risk for conditions that can cause SCA – including HCM. This questionnaire is available in several forms including hardcopy, online survey, and Facebook applications. It can be used in schools, recreation departments, houses of worship, the workplace, and places where young people and families gather. This is a one-directional questionnaire, which means it is not necessary or advised that the form be "turned in" to a central source. It is intended to inform the individual who is completing the form (for themselves or for a child) that they may wish to interact with their personal health-care provider and promote evaluation with a cardiologist. It provides step-by-step instructions on how to create this interplay with your physician. To download a copy of SCARAT, visit 4hcm.org.

The second community program that the HCMA supports focuses on cardiac emergencies and increasing response times and survival rates. The "Drill Dr. Heart" Program is geared toward preparing schools, athletic teams, and the workplace for cardiac emergencies. The first step is to assess each group's existing emergency action plans, or, if not already in place, to create one. The next step is to communicate this plan to the team, class, or workplace. Each emergency action plan is different and based on the individual setting and location of an AED. Once the plan is communicated, a drill is recommended to ensure that all parties understand the plan, permitting a proper and effective response to a cardiac emergency. To become involved with this program, contact the HCMA.

Driving

There are two different standards that apply to driving in the United States: commercial and personal. A diagnosis of HCM should have no bearing on a patient's personal driving privileges and license. If syncope (fainting) or near-syncope (near fainting) has been experienced, the physician may advise the patient not to drive until these symptoms can be better controlled and understood.

To obtain a commercial driver's license (CDL), there are specific fitness guidelines. These guidelines do change from time to time, and therefore you may want to consult the Department of Transportation (DOT) website for the latest information (www.fmcsa.dot.gov).

Currently, the CDL standard that is applied to HCM patients is found in the Cardiovascular Advisory Panel Guidelines for the Medical Examination of Commercial Motor Vehicle Drivers, FMCSA-MCP-02-002 October 2002, which specifically states the following:

> Irrespective of symptoms, a person should not be certified as a commercial driver if a firm diagnosis of HCM is made on echocardiography.

The DOT website section § 391.41 addresses the physical qualifications for drivers and was updated as of August 31, 2012. Section 391.41 (b) (4) specifically states the following: "Has no current clinical diagnosis of myocardial infarction, angina pectoris, coronary insufficiency, thrombosis, or any other cardiovascular disease of a variety known to be accompanied by syncope, dyspnea, collapse, or congestive cardiac failure." This statement could (and probably does) exclude patients with HCM.

There is also an appeal process, and with a favorable evaluation from a cardiologist, it may be possible to eventually obtain a CDL. Reevaluation is required annually, and a repetitive appeal process may be necessary. Therefore, we do not advise careers in this field for patients with HCM.

If you cannot walk long distances without symptoms such as shortness of breath, chest pain, or lightheadedness, it is suggested you apply for a handicapped parking permit. It is advised that patients who even occasionally have such symptoms request the handicapped parking permit as it is difficult to predict a "bad day" in advance. In many cases, this only involves a simple form that can be obtained from your local motor vehicle office (but must be signed by your doctor).

If you have an implantable defibrillator, consult with your cardiologist regarding local regulations governing automobile driving with these devices. In several states, it is suggested that defibrillator patients should not drive for up to 6 months after their implant. At this time, there does not appear to be a law governing this, and it is simply a recommendation. You and your physician should discuss your individual situation and decide what is in your best interest.

Traveling

You need to think about your health before you plan a trip. Remember to bring all medications with you and it is always a good idea to keep a letter in your possession explaining your medical condition. In US airports, you can ask for assistance to be transported to your gate; foreign airports vary greatly and you should ask your travel agent to make arrangements for you.

For those who are more symptomatic, it is critical to remember the importance of pacing yourself while on vacation, or you may become fatigued and will not enjoy yourself. Call ahead to see how far away the attractions are that you wish to see, and if necessary arrange for a motorized scooter or wheelchair.

Commercial airline travel itself (at altitudes conventionally involved) poses no risk to HCM patients. Caution should be exercised in scheduling vacations or trips to remote destinations where the level of medical care is rudimentary and where specific knowledge of HCM may be virtually nonexistent. The same considerations apply to traveling on cruise ships where the level of medical care may not be consistent and, in some instances, suboptimal for a patient with HCM. If you have an implantable defibrillator and are planning a trip, you may want to contact your electrophysiologist (or the device manufacturer) to identify the nearest suitable hospital to your vacation/business destination.

Customer service:

Medtronic, Inc.	1 800 633-8766 (USA)
710 Medtronic Parkway	1 763 514 4000 (USA)
Minneapolis, MN 55432-5604, USA	www.medtronic.com
Boston Scientific (formerly Guidant Corporation)	1 800 227 3422 (USA)
4100 Hamline Avenue North	1 651 582 4000 (USA)
St. Paul, MN 55112-5798, USA	www.bostonscientific.com
St. Jude Medical, Inc.	1 800 328 9634
One St. Jude Medical Drive	1 651 756 2000
St. Paul MN 55117-9913, USA	www.SJM.com
Biotronik	1 800-547-0394
6024 Jean Road	
Lake Oswego CA, 97035-5571	www.biotronik.com

Military service

Careers in the military are not encouraged for those with HCM for a variety of reasons. However, if you wish to pursue this career path, you should be aware of the following. As a general guideline, the military will disqualify any person with "hypertrophy" or "dilation" of the heart. If a person with HCM wishes to enter the military, there is an appeal process in which a petition can be made to the Service Waive Authorities for reevaluation. If a person has long-term disease stability, a waiver may be awarded. However, due to the variable nature of HCM, it is unlikely that such a waiver would be awarded. If HCM is knowingly misrepresented at recruitment or service entry, and is established later, that person will be removed from the military and possibly prosecuted.

For those currently serving in the military, many factors are evaluated in determining whether a person with any newly discovered medical condition may remain on active service. Several issues will be considered in the case of a new HCM diagnosis including (but not limited to) length of service, job assignment, and qualifications. If someone is early in their career, it is unlikely that the military will retain that person, who may then wish to apply for military disability. Military disability will pay a portion of your wages, but is not equivalent to Social Security Disability. The intent of military disability is, in most cases, to return that person to civilian life where employment will be available.

If the person is to remain in the military (and may already have an extensive career), it is likely that an assessment of the specific job functions can be requested. If that person is "fit for duty," they may remain in their assignment. If not, a new position and revised training program may be provided. However, with increasing frequency, the military is attempting to ensure – for matters of public safety, but also in the best interest of soldiers with a disease such as HCM – that recruits are Worldwide Qualified. This means that person must be able to work in any place the military may send them, without consideration for the availability of specific or specialized medical treatment. For example, if a person has an ICD and is stationed in a remote area, would the military be able to provide the necessary care to ensure that person's health and well-being?

The Americans with Disabilities Act does not provide protection for those in the US Military. If you live outside of the United States, you should check with your local military recruitment center to inquire with the military guidelines in your country.

Social security benefits

Those in the United States who have severe limitation in daily-life functions because of their HCM may be eligible for Social Security Disability Insurance (SSI) coverage. However, a diagnosis of HCM is not itself sufficient to claim disability under SSI. Social Security defines "disability" as the inability to do any kind of work for which you are suited or trained: your disability is expected to last for at least 1 year.

The definition of disability under Social Security is different than in other programs. Social Security pays for only total disability. No benefits are payable for partial or for short-term disability. Disability under Social

Security is based on the inability to work. You are considered disabled under Social Security rules if you cannot perform work that you did before and Social Security decides that you cannot adjust to other employment because of your medical condition(s). Social Security program rules also assume that working families have access to other resources to provide support during periods of short-term disabilities, including workers' compensation, insurance, savings, and investments.

You may receive Social Security Disability benefits at any age. If you are receiving such benefits at age 65 years, that amount will become your retirement benefit. Your dependents may be eligible for additional Social Security insurance benefits if your household income is low enough to create financial need. They include

- Your unmarried children, including stepchildren, adopted children, or, in some cases, grandchildren, under the age of 18 years (or 19 years if still a full-time high school student).
- Your unmarried child, 18 years or older, if your disability started before the age of 22 years.
- Your spouse if 62 years or older, or any age if he or she is caring for a child of yours who is under 16 years or disabled, and is also receiving disability checks.
- Your disabled widow or widower 50 years or older. The disability must have occurred before your death or within 7 years after your death.
- Your disabled ex-wife or ex-husband who is 50 years or older, if marriage lasted at least 10 years.

Your local Social Security office will send your application to the Disability Determination Service (DDS) office in your state. A team consisting of a physician (or psychologist) and a disability evaluation specialist will consider all facts and decide if you are "disabled" by their definition. They determine whether you can perform work-related activities such as walking, sitting, lifting, and carrying. Social Security benefits are also available to the surviving children of those who have died of HCM if the parent had worked in the United States. You should contact your local Social Security Administration (SSA) office to apply for benefits.

If your claim is denied, there are four levels of appeal available. As this is a complicated process, many choose to have an attorney represent them. To secure a lawyer, contact your local Bar Association for the names of disability attorneys in your area. For more information on Social Security, call them directly at 800 772 1213. A very useful area of the SSA website is http://www.ssa.gov/disabiltiy/professionals/bluebook/4.00-Cardiovascular-Adult.htm.

Family and Medical Leave Act

The Family and Medical Leave Act (FMLA) became effective in 1993. The purpose of this Act is to help balance the demands of the workplace with the needs of families by allowing eligible employees to take up to 12 weeks of unpaid, job-protected leave (during any 12-month period) for specific family emergencies such as serious illness or the birth of a child. Employers who have 50 or more employees working 20 or more weeks in the current or preceding calendar year and who are engaged in commerce are covered as well as public agencies (including governmental agencies and schools). To be eligible an employee must have worked

1 For a covered employer for at least 12 months.
2 At least 1250 hours during the past 12 months; at a location where at least 50 other employees are living within 75 miles of the workplace.

Many states have their own version of FMLA that run in conjunction with the Federal program. For specific information about FMLA in your state, check with the State Department of Labor.

Health insurance

We are living in a time of change in the world of insurance coverage under the Affordable Care Act. These reforms have given Americans new rights and benefits by helping more children get health coverage, ending lifetime and most annual limits on care, allowing young adults under 26 to stay on their parent's health insurance, and giving patients access to recommended preventive services without cost. Regardless of health-care reform, the basics will remain much the same with your policy options dictated by your employer. This is how the overwhelming majority of Americans access health insurance.

Your choice of health insurance can have a dramatic effect on the level of health care you receive. In the United States, most people are insured through employer-based programs in which individuals are given options to review on an annual basis.

Health Maintenance Organizations (HMOs) are normally the least expensive in terms of premiums, but also have the most restrictions and are often difficult to navigate if you are living with an uncommon condition like HCM. HMOs often claim to have doctors within their network who can evaluate your HCM; however, these doctors are often general cardiologists with no specific expertise in HCM. In general, HMOs are not the best option for patients with HCM.

Preferred Provider Organizations (PPOs) allow for in-and-out of network care and normally have premiums that are reasonable. PPOs allow the patient to seek out care with the most experienced centers and, in most cases, the major HCM Centers participate with many large health-care carrier "plans," thus keeping patients "in network." However, in the event you fall "out of network," you would have to pay a deductible in order to receive care in an experienced center, unlike HMOs who can refuse to pay any portion of the claim.

Point of Service (POS) plans can be difficult to understand as some have "referral required" clauses which make them more like a disguised HMO. However, if the POS has no referral required, it will, in most cases, act like a PPO.

Traditional indemnity plans are making a comeback and are a very good option as they simply provide coverage on a percentage split, 80% paid by the insurance carrier and 20% by the patient up to an out-of-pocket maximum of a set amount. These plans allow for the greatest freedom and are priced rather competitively.

Patients may meet financial criteria for state-subsidized health care, Medicaid, which will provide some coverage. In the event the patient is qualified for Social Security either based on age or disability, they may qualify for Medicare, in which case purchasing a Medicare supplement is advised.

The Health Insurance Portability and Accountability Act of 1996 (HIPAA) set forth the federal rules for preexisting medical conditions. Under HIPAA, preexisting conditions must be covered by a new plan as long as the participant has maintained some form of coverage without a break of 63 days. This means you can leave one job and start a new one without the plan disqualifying coverage for HCM treatment (as long as you have not broken coverage for 63 days). You may need to purchase Consolidated Omnibus Budget Reconciliation Act (COBRA) coverage to protect you in such circumstances.

Life insurance

While the diagnosis of HCM will not always leave you "uninsurable," it may nevertheless result in very high premiums. You must also disclose all medical information to the insurance company. With this in mind, it may be a wise idea to purchase coverage prior to being screened for HCM. If you have already been diagnosed with HCM, you can purchase coverage from a number of "assigned risk" carriers. A better idea is to maximize any group insurance your employer, credit card company, or civic organization may offer.

Coverage for children may be taken as a "rider" on an existing adult policy. These provisions are in most cases "nonmedical," which means that no medical questions are asked regarding the child. Many such "riders" can be converted to a separate policy at age 18 years, and at as much as five times the original value. This is a good way to ensure coverage for the child into adulthood.

State laws govern life insurance, so it is important to contact your local independent insurance broker to advise you of the best options for your family. Remember, when speaking to the agent, you are not required to disclose all important information when shopping for insurance. When completing the application, it is also important not to disclose the medical information of others, but be more general in nature. Those seeking genetic testing should remember that while Genetic Information Nondiscrimination Act (GINA) provides protection for health insurance, it offers no protection for life insurance. Thus, it is important to secure some life insurance *before* clinical genetic testing.

Students

During the education process, children and young adults with HCM may face obstacles related to their diagnosis or treatment. It is advised to put in place (in the United States) a 504 Plan, which offers the student a level of protection and accommodation. A "504 Plan" refers to the Section 504 of the *Rehabilitation Act* and the *Americans with Disabilities Act* which specifies that no one with a disability can be excluded from participating in federally funded programs or activities, including elementary, secondary, or postsecondary schooling. "Disability" in this context refers to a "physical or mental impairment which substantially limits one or more major life activities." This can include physical impairments; illnesses or injuries; communicable diseases; chronic conditions like HCM. A 504 Plan spells out modifications and accommodations that will be needed for these students to have an opportunity to perform at the same level as their peers, and might include such things as additional time to pass from class to class, alternative gym activities, additional time for standardize testing (due to medication side effects), an extra set of textbooks, home instruction, or a tape recorder in class. It may also include the direction for an AED to be available at the school for the child. Because the Americans with Disabilities Act is a federal law, all states must comply, yet some districts seem more willing to do so than others.

The HCMA offers a sample 504 on its website which can be used as a template.

HCM Centers

The concept of an HCM Center is to provide patients with a clinical environment separate from general cardiology in which they are in contact with health-care professionals focused and dedicated to their disease, in which all treatment options are available. This is in recognition that HCM is different from the more common coronary artery disease with its own strategies for diagnosis and treatment. Cardiologists involved in such centers have in fact made a commitment to HCM that is clearly in the best interests of the patient population.

The first such centers were probably at the National Institutes of Health (NIH), at Toronto General Hospital, and in Sydney, Australia, although the NIH program was terminated due to government scandal. The center in Sydney, Australia, initially directed by Dr. David Richmond was the first in a medical school/university setting and continues to this day. Twenty years ago, an HCM program was organized at the Minneapolis Heart Institute, followed by the Mayo Clinic and Tufts Medical Center, and now there are many more. Over the last 15 years, the HCMA has worked in concert with cardiologists to promote such programs with more than 20 HCM Centers currently established, although somewhat variable in size and experience. These centers allow HCM patients access to the optimal care in environments with high HCM patient volume, and which are often relatively close to their home and local cardiologists. Visiting an HCM Center does not exclude the care provided by your local cardiologist, as the two are designed to work together in the best interests of the patients.

- Patients with HCM should maintain a consistent relationship with a local area cardiologist, but optimally also have regular input from an HCM program.
- Programs at HCM Centers are generally preferred for major treatment interventions and risk assessment.

Support and advocacy groups (HCMA)

"Support groups" take a variety of forms, including those confined to the family unit and close friends. As individuals, however, we often find the need to discuss the unique issues and problems, or find answers to complex questions that our family or friends may not be able to provide.

Such has been the substrate for creating support or advocacy groups focused on specific (often uncommon) medical conditions. Previously, such patient and disease-related support organizations were uncommon and located largely in local communities for the purpose of meeting directly to discuss common problems and sharing insights. This format allowed each person to seek the support of others affected by the same life circumstances they had experienced. The advent of the Internet has created an easier, inexpensive, and instantaneous free flow of information and contact between the interested parties, in the context of online support groups, independent of geography, or even international boundaries. This more efficient dissemination of information has made a substantial difference for patients with uncommon diseases such as HCM. The HCMA was at the forefront of the movement using the Internet for patient advocacy by establishing its first website in 1996 and its first community message board in 2000.

Most physicians understand the need for and benefits of support groups. Furthermore, many studies have shown that a positive attitude toward chronic disease has a direct influence on the patient's quality of life. Support groups offer patients and families the information and foundation with which they can deal more effectively with their medical condition. In addition to a better quality of life for the patient, the entire family will benefit from a clearer understanding of the chronic disease (which in many cases is familial). The clarity achieved from the support group will also help patients communicate effectively with physicians.

The HCMA was founded in 1996 by Lisa Salberg in the memory of her sister, Lori Anne Flanigan, who (although diagnosed years earlier) died suddenly of HCM. It was the aspiration of the founder to help others with HCM to have a complete and unbiased understanding of their disease, and to provide a window (and access) to all available treatment options free from institutional bias and consistent with current medical literature and societal guidelines and recommendations.

Indeed, one of the key elements of the HCMA is the facilitation of appropriate and accurate information by interfacing the patient (who is often confused about his or her disease) directly with medical literature or clinicians who are experts in HCM. Frequently, patients with HCM are confused by the hard-core medical scientific literature, which can also promote exaggerated pessimism, or by a limited familiarity with HCM to which their local cardiologist or internist may readily concede.

However, technological advances have dramatically changed that state of affairs by substantially enhancing and embracing communication, thereby offering HCM patients the opportunity to quickly become appropriately informed regarding the nature and implications of their disease. In addition to such free flow of information via the Internet, the HCMA sponsors a national meeting in New Jersey, and regional meetings throughout the United States, which bring patients, families, clinical cardiologists, and researchers together to interact in a unique environment of partnership.

The HCMA's vision statement embodies our aspirations, as the preeminent organization dedicated to improving the lives of those with HCM, preventing untimely death, and advancing global understanding. The mission statement describes our focus: providing support, advocacy, and education to patients, families, the medical community, and the public about HCM while fostering research and innovation.

The specific goals and objectives of the HCMA are
- To develop and maintain a network of support for people with HCM, their families, and the medical community.
- To promote education about the symptoms, risks, and treatment options to those living with HCM, as well as access to expert professional care.
- To raise awareness of protection against sudden death.
- To develop and maintain a network of health-care providers knowledgeable about the diagnosis and treatment of HCM.
- To promote research in HCM, and provide ready access to this information.

The HCMA provides a vast number of services to its membership including, but not limited to
- Intimate, regionally located, person-to-person meetings
- Emotional support to individual patients and families with HCM
- Information about, and access to, medical providers
- Education to patients and the medical practitioners and community advocacy
- Internet-based access, including a message board
- International contacts to further the interests of its members

The HCMA also provides individual confidential support for matters related to
- Concerns over a recent diagnosis
- Questions regarding "centers of excellence" in the field of HCM
- Information about all aspects of HCM and its treatment options
- Support to families who may have lost a relative or friend to HCM
- Access to other HCM patients with whom they share a unique bond

The HCMA provides those with HCM (or their family members) with the ability to make direct contact with other HCM patients. When you have been diagnosed with such a genetic disorder, which is relatively uncommon in cardiology practices, access to other patients with the same disease provides a sense of belonging and the assurance that you are not alone.

Other international HCM Support Groups that you may contact:

In the United Kingdom

The Cardiomyopathy Association www.cardiomyopathy.org
Unit 10 Chiltern Court
Asheridge Road Tel: 01494 791 224
Chesham Bucks, HP5 2PX UK Fax: 01494 797 199

In Australia and New Zealand

Cardiomyopathy Association of
Australia Ltd.
P.O Box 273
Hurstbridge, Victoria 3099, Australia

www.CMAA.org.au
Tel: 144 1300 552 622
Fax: 144 03 9499 1687

In Ireland

Irish Heart Foundation
50 Ringsend Rd
Dublin 4, Ireland

www.irishheart.ie
Tel: 1353 1 6685001
Fax: 1353 1 6685896

In Israel

The Israeli hypertrophic
Cardiomyopathy Association

giead.org.il/ihcma/
Tel: 1972 03 629 9389

In Italy

Azienda Ospedaliera Universitara Careggi
Largo Brambilia 3
50134, Firenze, Italy

www.aou-careggi.toscana.it
39 055 794 111

For those who have had or will have cardiac surgery:

The Mended Hearts, Inc.
8150 N. Central Expressway, M2248
Dallas, Texas 75206

www.mendedhearts.org
Tel: 1-888-HEART99
Email: info@mendedhearts.org

What research is being conducted?

Research is a critical aspect of the future of HCM, yet is rarely discussed with patients. Nevertheless, patients are encouraged to participate in research protocols with proper institutional oversight and solid medical science. In most instances, patients fulfill this aspiration simply by permitting their clinical data to be shared in institutional databases. There are currently several vigorous HCM research programs largely in the United States, Canada, Europe, and Japan. The most important and relevant research efforts emphasize further definition and clarification of the diagnostic features and clinical course of HCM, particularly with respect to novel treatment strategies; for example, the application of the ICD to HCM has changed the course of the disease for many patients. Also, research aimed at identifying and characterizing the gene mutations that cause HCM is being performed in selected laboratories in the United States, largely in Mayo Clinic and Brigham and Women's Hospital.

There are several US centers with long-term commitments to clinical research in HCM. These include Minneapolis Heart Institute, Tufts Medical Center (Boston), Mayo Clinic, St. Luke's Roosevelt Medical Center (New York), and Brigham and Women's Hospital (Boston). However, as is the case with many relatively uncommon diseases, a limited number of clinical research grants are available specifically for HCM. Consequently, financial support for HCM research continues to be sparse and sporadic, coming largely from private foundations and industry, but rarely from NIH or AHA sources.

The US Government has strict guidelines and safeguards to protect patients in research studies. Research that involves human subjects must be approved and monitored by an Institutional Review Board (IRB). The IRB assures that potential risks are as low as possible and are clearly explained to participants to enable a fully informed decision.

Before you are allowed to participate in a study, you will be asked to sign an "informed consent." "Informed consent" is the process of learning the key facts about a study before you decide whether or not to participate. While some people may see this as a simple administrative step, you should nevertheless carefully review these documents so that you fully understand the study and your commitment. It is also important to remember that declining participation will not have adverse consequences on your care with your treating doctor. We encourage patients to stay in touch with the HCMA to learn of upcoming research opportunities.

The 36 most frequently asked questions about HCM that are addressed to the HCMA by patients, caregivers, and family members

1 *How did I get HCM?*
HCM is a genetic disease; therefore you are born with the genetic code to develop HCM. You may not have developed symptoms that indicate that you have HCM, but nevertheless you are indeed born with an abnormal gene. However, what actually triggers the mutation to occur is unknown and environmental factors could conceivably play a role at that point. It is also unknown exactly how the mutation in your DNA causes the heart to be abnormal and create HCM.

2 *Will my heart get bigger?*
After reaching full maturity, normally by age 18–20 years, your heart growth usually stops. There are occasional exceptions, as in "adult-onset" hypertrophy. However, this rule covers an estimated 90–95% of the relevant clinical situations. You should not be concerned that your heart will grow perpetually – that is, increase thickness throughout life, as there is always a point at which growth and thickening of the heart stops.

3 *I thought it was good to have big muscles, so what is wrong with a thick heart muscle?*
Having "big" muscles may sound like a good thing to some. However, an abnormally thick heart muscle is not beneficial to your health, particularly if the thickening creates a situation in which the heart cannot properly fill with blood during the relaxation phase (diastole), or increases the risk for important arrhythmias when extreme, such as may occur in HCM.

4 *I get very tired or notice more chest discomfort after a big meal. Is this normal or is it my HCM?*

This is a very common complaint among HCM patients. There is, in fact, some evidence that a heavy meal can increase outflow obstruction and shortness of breath in HCM. We suggest you eat smaller meals and try to avoid heavy foods. You will also want to avoid fatty and greasy foods and eating late at night.

5 *I've had symptoms of dizziness, chest pain, and sometimes I'm short of breath. I don't like to complain to my cardiologist. When should I call him or her about my symptoms?*
You should discuss your symptoms, in as much detail as appropriate, with your cardiologist at your regular visits. Establish with your cardiologist how to communicate new symptoms or increased frequency of your symptoms. If new symptoms are pronounced, you should contact your physician. Most HCM-related symptoms can be addressed in a cardiologist's office and emergency room visits are infrequent.

6 *Should I have children?*
This is an issue of genetic counseling and does not lend itself easily to a yes or no answer, but is largely a matter of individual choice. It is a very common question for both men and women to confront at some point in their life. HCM is an autosomal-dominant disease, which means it is transmitted to about 50% of each consecutive generation. Therefore, a child born to a patient with HCM has a statistical 50:50 chance of inheriting the family mutation for HCM. However, it is important to remember that most people with HCM live normal lives without significant disability or the necessity for major medical interventions. Therefore, genetic counseling rarely advises against having children, although in those families with multiple sudden deaths or particularly serious disease manifestations, consideration should be given to not propagating what is obviously a malignant disease process.

Women with HCM usually experience normal pregnancies, and there are no data suggesting that it is generally harmful to be pregnant with HCM. In some cases, women can remain on certain heart medication during the entire pregnancy (your obstetrician must be consulted on this point). Delivery may very occasionally convey an added risk in selected patients with HCM. Epidural anesthesia has been associated with complications such as low blood pressure, and therefore we suggest that you discuss this strategy with your obstetrician and anesthesiologist well before delivery. If you choose to become pregnant, you may also want to discuss breast-feeding with your doctor to ensure that your medications will not adversely affect your baby.

7 *Can I exercise? What type of recreational activities or sports can I participate in and what should I avoid?*

The majority of patients with HCM can participate in moderate exercise and in fact are encouraged to be physically active. Walking, lap swimming, skating, bowling, bicycle riding, golf, archery, yoga, and tai-chi are examples of activities in which you may feel comfortable participating. You should consult with your cardiologist to tailor the most appropriate recreational exercise program to ensure that you are not unnecessarily placing yourself at risk.

Particularly discouraged are those activities involving "burst" exertion in which the heart rate increases abruptly such as sprinting, or any sports activity which creates circumstances in which individuals cannot use their best judgment to stop and withdraw. Consider that the onset of a given sensation (e.g., lightheadedness) could, in fact, represent an HCM-related symptom, and not simply a consequence of intense athletic activity. Finally, patients should avoid physical activities which provoke symptoms such as shortness of breath, chest pain, lightheadedness, or syncope. Helpful AHA guidelines for recreational sports activities are presented in this book in Table 3.

8 *Will HCM affect my sex life?*

HCM, as well as some medications used to treat the disease, can cause fatigue, so there may be a lack of energy rather than an absence of interest in sex. However, medications used to treat HCM, such as beta-blockers, can occasionally cause impotence. In general, patients with HCM should be able to enjoy a normal and active sex life. If you feel that either your medications or your diagnosis is having an adverse impact on your sex life, you should have an open and frank discussion with your cardiologist. Alternative medications may be available. This question is the one that tends to cause the most unnecessary stress for patients and their partners. In general, patients with HCM should be able to enjoy a normal sex life.

9 *I have thought about taking medications for erectile dysfunction such as Viagra. Are there any risks specifically for HCM patients?*

There are theoretical risks, since such drugs may cause or worsen obstruction. However, there have been no documented adverse events in HCM. Therefore, you should consult your cardiologist before starting or continuing on this class of medication.

10 *Should I seek out an HCM specialist? How do I know if someone is an HCM specialist?*
The HCMA recommends that patients with HCM consult at some time with a cardiologist who specializes in HCM. Routine annual visits seem to work best in a chronic disease such as HCM, whether or not the patient perceives any clinical interval change. This may involve some travel because there are relatively few such cardiologists who have focused their professional energy on this disease. Although it is not always convenient to travel to an HCM specialist or center, in many cases such a strategy has made a substantial difference in the quality of care our HCMA members have received. It is also imperative to work with your hometown (local) cardiologist and keep the lines of communication open between all parties. An optimal situation is one in which your care involves both a knowledgeable local cardiologist and an HCM Center. The HCMA keeps a registry of all cardiologists who have either a special interest or experience with HCM, and are well respected by their peers.

11 *Should I tell my cousins, aunts, uncles, or blood relatives that I have been diagnosed with HCM?*
Yes, because HCM is a genetic disease. Although it may be difficult to talk about this, you are obligated to let your family know. All blood relatives should be screened for HCM (with echocardiography, ECG, probably cardiac MRI, and consultation with a cardiologist), particularly if there have been premature deaths due to heart disease in the family. The HCMA can assist in such communication to your extended family.

12 *Sometimes I think I am depressed. It is hard living with a chronic disease. What can I do to feel better?*
Do not be afraid to discuss your feelings with your physician. Depression can be a consequence of how you perceive your life situation, or possibly a side effect of a cardiac drug. Therefore, you may need to change medications to help relieve your depression. Whether or not a drug reaction is causing your depression, it might be prudent to see a

psychiatrist, psychologist, or another mental health clinician to discuss your feelings. Certainly, living with a chronic disease *is* difficult and you should not hesitate to seek help in dealing with the emotional component of the condition. In families where there has been a death related to HCM, and other family members also have HCM, family/ group counseling may prove helpful. Hopefully, some of the ideas in this book, and the HCMA website (www.4HCM.org) will be useful.

13 *I live in a remote area, the local hospital is very small, and I am afraid they will not know how to help me. What can I do to help them help me?*

Take a proactive role in your own health care. While AEDs are rather common today, contact your local ambulance service and see if they have an AED and confirm response times to your home. If the response time is more than 3 minutes on average, you may want to consider an AED for your home. If you are not seen to be at "high risk" for SCA it is not likely this will be needed. However, if you live in a rural area, it seems wise to stop and think about the issue. In addition, you may want to stop by the local emergency room and bring them information (such as in this book). By doing this, you will provide those health-care workers with the opportunity to understand HCM and your particular situation better, so that they will be ready for you in case you need them. The HCMA provides emergency information cards for patients to carry; please contact our office to obtain one. You may also request HCMA to provide an information kit to your hospital or the physician's office. Simply e-mail the name and address of the health-care provider to support@4HCM.org.

14 *Are there any other conditions that cause HCM, or can HCM cause any other conditions?*

There are syndromes that have been associated with a thick left ventricular wall closely resembling HCM. These conditions are not really HCM, but appear similar, including storage diseases which are metabolic conditions. For example, Danon disease (LAMP2) is such a disorder, which differs distinctly from typical HCM by virtue of being a metabolic storage disease. Also, Noonan syndrome is associated with a thick heart muscle (but it differs in its genetic basis from HCM).

15 *Is it usual to feel tired because of HCM?*

Yes, fatigue is probably the most common complaint we hear at the HCMA; however, it is a symptom which is distinctive from shortness of breath occurring with physical exertion. The basis for fatigue in HCM is not well understood. Some fatigue may be related to medications given for HCM; therefore it is important to talk to your cardiologist about such symptoms and see what can be done to try to minimize them – this may include a switch in medications. In addition, there is some evidence that a heavy meal can accentuate outflow obstruction in HCM and therefore symptoms such as shortness of breath. We suggest you eat smaller meals and try to avoid heavy foods. You will also want to avoid eating late at night.

16 *Can I drink caffeine? Eat salt?*
You should consult with your physician for specific dietary restrictions and needs. Caffeine can have adverse reactions in some people and cause a racing heart. Therefore, if you are prone to arrhythmias, you may want to avoid excessive caffeine. Keep in mind that there are substantial amounts of caffeine in products other than coffee, such as Coca-Cola®, tea, energy drinks, and chocolate. Excessive salt (sodium) may be harmful to those with high blood pressure or heart failure. If you are experiencing heart failure symptoms, excessive amounts of sodium should be avoided.

17 *How important is my cholesterol level?*
Just because you have HCM does not mean you are at any less risk for other forms of cardiovascular disease. Some people with HCM also have high blood pressure and/or coronary artery disease due to atherosclerosis (mostly over age 50). Therefore, it is always a good idea to keep a "healthy heart" diet. On the other hand, HCM is not protective in any way against atherosclerosis. The principle is to keep your heart as healthy as you can to avoid having the additional burden of a second, or even a third condition.

18 *Why can't they just cut my heart "down to size"?*
This is not the answer to this disease. It would be medically untenable to remove enough abnormal muscle by surgery, or any other means, to "cure" a complex condition such as HCM. Even if that were possible, normalizing the heart structure would not necessarily solve the overall problem, since the portions of the heart wall with normal thickness may also have abnormal function. Of note, the myectomy operation does, by design, remove a portion of muscle from the ventricular septum. However, the surgeon only resects a small amount of tissue (i.e., 2–6 g) in hearts where the usual overall weight is about 500 g or more.

19 *Can I drink alcohol?*

Yes, in moderation. There are few data on the effects of alcohol consumption in HCM, but moderation is advised. Alcohol can also have a depressant effect on heart muscle function. Furthermore, consumption of even a small amount of alcohol has been shown to increase the degree of obstruction and symptoms, by acting as a stimulant.

20 *What effect will marijuana have on someone with HCM?*

There is no direct evidence regarding this drug in patients with HCM. Nevertheless, it is conservative (and prudent) to avoid marijuana. In addition, this drug increases the rate and force of heart contractions. This could place a substantial burden on the HCM heart, especially with long-term use.

21 *What effect will the use of cocaine, heroin, or methamphetamines have on someone with HCM?*

Although their precise actions with respect to HCM are not known with certainty, the use of these "recreational" drugs could prove adverse in someone with a complex disease such as HCM, and should be avoided absolutely. All of these drugs release metabolites which persistently increase heart rate and blood pressure. Cocaine itself can be responsible for heart attacks and sudden cardiac death due to inflammation of the heart muscle and weakening of the walls of the coronary arteries.

22 *Can I become a pilot?*

In the United States, a commercial pilot must pass a physical examination annually for the Federal Aviation Administration (FAA). Awarding a nonrestricted first-class commercial license to a pilot with HCM is a controversial issue which may be associated with substantial administrative difficulties. At present, it is often possible to obtain a third-class (private aircraft) license with HCM.

23 *Are there any occupations I should avoid?*

If possible, you should probably avoid occupations that predominantly require particularly strenuous physical labor, and long distance or public safety-related driving. In some HCM patients, intense physical activity undertaken chronically could prove detrimental, by conceivably raising your arrhythmia and sudden death risk. In addition, if you have an implanted device (pacemaker/defibrillator), you will need to avoid certain occupations such as those requiring contact with transmitting antennas and their power source, diathermy equipment (found in hospitals), power transmission lines, and electrical equipment (such as for welding).

24 *Is a cure coming soon?*
You should not expect or anticipate HCM to be "cured." HCM is a complex, chronic disease, but one which is managed or controlled in many ways, and should be regarded as treatable. Major advances such as the implantable defibrillator may alter the natural history of the disease for many patients and restore an opportunity for normal or near-normal longevity. Although we have made great strides in identifying the genes that cause HCM, a cure (such as with gene therapy) is not a reasonable aspiration due to the extremely complex and challenging scientific issues involved.

25 *Can my child participate in competitive sports?*
Generally, no. Young patients with HCM are discouraged from participating in most intense competitive sports. There have been three national cardiology conferences (known as the Bethesda Conferences) over the last 20 years which have consistently made this recommendation. Notable exceptions to these exclusions are competitive golf, and bowling (both with growing sports traditions in high school). This may be a very difficult adjustment for both parent and child. Of note, there is no other clinical circumstance in HCM management that has the same capacity for emotion and misunderstanding (and sometimes anger) as the recommendation to disqualify young athletes from competitive sports because of HCM.

26 *Can my child participate in gym class?*
If the child is capable of participating in basic activities, the school doctor or nurse may work with the physical education teacher to tailor a realistic program. In some school systems, this is called adaptive physical education. However, for most children with HCM, this question arises without symptoms. Therefore, you and the school should recognize that certain gym class sports activities may be intense and truly competitive in nature – for example, the traditional 600 yard run for time – and such physical activity should be avoided. It is most important to work these matters out prospectively and directly with the school, and in detail. You may want to consult a 504 Plan for your child.

27 *Can I SCUBA dive?*
There is no information available that would suggest that the act of self-contained underwater breathing apparatus (SCUBA) diving itself creates physiologic alterations which are dangerous to HCM patients. However, SCUBA is usually a paired activity requiring submersion with a partner. Therefore, any impairment in consciousness, incapacitation, or onset of symptoms (due to HCM) would also unavoidably impact the safety of another person. For these reasons, this particular sporting activity is probably not advisable for patients with HCM.

28 *Why is HCM more common and worse in men?*
Actually, it is not. HCM is an autosomal-dominant genetic trait, and therefore it occurs equally in men and women. However, it is obvious that HCM is recognized clinically much more commonly in men (about 60:40), suggesting that for a variety of reasons this disease is underdiagnosed in women. In addition, heart failure is diagnosed later in women and may be more severe at that time. However, there is no gender difference with respect to likelihood of sudden death. Sudden death due to HCM in young athletes is significantly more common in males than in females.

29 *Are there additional problems that can occur from dehydration in HCM?*
Patients with HCM can have significant increase in symptoms when dehydrated, often due to the onset of obstruction or an increase in its severity. Therefore, patients should be careful to maintain proper hydration by drinking adequate fluids on a daily basis.

30 *In the event of an emergency, should I or my family inform emergency service workers of my HCM diagnosis?*
Absolutely, you should inform the emergency room that you have HCM. You should also be aware that HCM patients sometimes have ECGs that appear to suggest that a myocardial infarction ("heart attack") has occurred. Furthermore, you should inform the emergency personnel that nitroglycerine (a drug administered to "heart attack" victims) may aggravate chest pain/angina and other symptoms in HCM patients, and can also cause a severe drop in blood pressure and promote obstruction, which can be dangerous to unstable HCM patients.

31 *Should I apply for disability if I have HCM?*
No, not solely because you have HCM. However, you may want to consider this strategy if your symptoms limit your ability to function in

the workplace. Disability is not granted based on diagnosis; it is justified with respect to limits in functional capacity.

32 *Isn't alcohol ablation an "easy" technique with little risk, at least compared to surgery?*
In reality, the risks of myectomy surgery in an experienced center are somewhat *less* than those for ablation. For example, there have been zero reported myectomy-related deaths over the last decade at surgical centers such as Mayo Clinic, Cleveland Clinic, and Tufts Medical Center. There is also the concern that in some young patients alcohol ablation may increase risk for arrhythmias and sudden death over the long time period during which such individuals are exposed to unpredictable events.

33 *"Obstruction" sounds bad to me. Should I worry?*
Not necessarily. Obstruction to flow of blood out of the left ventricle is a pressure gradient between the left ventricle and the aorta which raises pressures within the left ventricular chamber. It should be emphasized that this term does not imply a total obstruction to flow, but only a partial one caused by the mitral valve moving forward to contact the ventricular septum during contraction in systole. Obstruction is very common in HCM; 70% of patients have it at rest or can generate it with exercise when the heart rate is elevated. *However, only some patients develop progressive symptoms and limitation due to obstruction requiring surgery (or alternatively alcohol ablation). Moreover, HCM Centers have many older patients in their sixties, seventies, and even eighties with obstruction, but without symptoms or the need for intervention.*

34 *What kind of health insurance should I have?*
Any insurance coverage is better than no coverage at all. If at all possible, HMOs should be avoided in favor of PPOs, POS (without referral required), or indemnity plans. Many states offer plans for children at attractive rates and you should contact your local health department or school for more information on these programs. If you meet the financial requirements within your state, you may be eligible for a state-subsidized program; they may have different names including Medicaid. If you are on federal disability or are eligible based on age for Social Security benefits, you likely qualify for Medicare health coverage. If you are on Medicare, it is advised that you also purchase a Medicare supplement.

35 *My child's school is holding a heart screening program. Can't I just have him checked there?*

No, community-based screening programs are not thorough enough for those from HCM families and in fact there are few data at this time to support the concept of community screenings with ECGs or limited echocardiography to detect HCM at all.

36 *Will genetic testing predict the course of my HCM?*

Genetic testing does not predict the precise clinical course for patients with HCM.

Glossary

This is a list of scientific terms commonly used with regard to HCM, defined in a relatively straightforward fashion, but avoiding medical jargon, as much as possible. Some of these terms are also defined in the text, and are repeated here for completeness.

Ambulatory: Refers to tests performed when a person performs their normal daily activities.

Angina: Chest pain or discomfort usually brought on by exertion and relieved by rest. Angina results from insufficient oxygen supply to the heart muscle.

Angiography: An X-ray of the heart and blood vessels obtained at the time of cardiac catheterization with the injection of contrast dye. This test may be performed to assess the anatomy of the coronary arteries (blood vessels which supply the heart muscle).

Anticoagulation: Treatment to reduce the potential of blood to form clots (e.g., with heparin or warfarin). Such treatment is employed when there is a risk of clot formation in the heart, such as in the atria associated with atrial fibrillation.

Aorta: The main blood vessel which arises from the left ventricle and carries blood from the heart to the rest of the body.

Apex: The bottom portion of the heart; the tip of the left ventricle.

Aneurysm: A bulging outward of the left ventricular wall due to thinning and scarring in that area.

A Guide to Hypertrophic Cardiomyopathy: For Patients, Their Families, and Interested Physicians, Third Edition. Barry J. Maron and Lisa Salberg.
© 2014 John Wiley & Sons, Ltd. Published 2014 by John Wiley & Sons, Ltd.

Arrhythmia: An abnormal rhythm or irregularity of the heartbeat. The heartbeat may either be too fast (*tachycardia*) or too slow (*bradycardia*). Arrhythmias may cause symptoms such as palpitations or lightheadedness or many have more serious consequences including sudden death.

Atria: The two filling chambers of the heart, one on the right and one on the left. Blood is collected in the atria while the ventricles are contracting. This blood is then released from the atria into the ventricles when they are ready to fill.

Atrial fibrillation: A common type of arrhythmia in which the atria loses its normal contraction pattern and the heart rhythm becomes irregular. Atrial fibrillation may be transient or persistent.

Cardiac arrest: When the heart ceases to have an effective rhythm and contraction, and death is imminent.

Cardiac catheterization: A special invasive test used in patients with many forms of heart disease, including selected patients with HCM. A fine tube (catheter) is passed from a blood vessel (in the arm or groin) into the heart, using X-ray guidance, and pressures within the heart chambers are measured. Heart structure and function can be assessed.

Cardiomyopathy: Refers to any disease predominantly involving the heart muscle; *cardia* refers to the heart and *myopathy* describes an abnormality of the heart muscle.

Concentric hypertrophy: The circumstance in which the left ventricular wall is thickened uniformly; also, referred to as symmetric hypertrophy. This is a rare pattern in HCM.

Congestive heart failure: A condition where weakness in the beating action of the heart causes fluid retention and symptoms of shortness of breath and fatigue on exercise. While this form of heart failure may occur in a few HCM patients with progressive disease, heart failure in HCM much more commonly occurs by a different mechanism related to the impaired relaxation and filling of the ventricles in diastole (and in the presence of normal beating action of the heart).

Coronary artery disease: The common condition in which the coronary arteries (that deliver blood to the heart muscle) are narrowed by the accumulation of fatty plaque. When clots form on these plaques, a "heart attack" (myocardial infarction) may result.

Diastole: Relaxation phase of the heart cycle when the ventricles passively fill with blood.

Diuretics: Drugs which increase the production of urine by the kidneys and decrease fluid retention.

Dominant inheritance: A disease which is transmitted to each consecutive generation and occurs in about 50% of the relatives in a generation.

Echocardiogram (commonly shortened to **echo**): Echocardiography is the single most important test in the assessment of HCM. This is a noninvasive ultrasound scan of the heart, which produces an image of the chambers, walls, and valves that can be viewed as a real-time movie (and is recorded permanently on videotape). *Doppler ultrasound* is part of the echocardiographic examination and produces a color-coded image of blood flow within the heart, detects areas of turbulent flow, and accurately measures the degree of obstruction. The pattern of filling of the left ventricle can also be assessed.

Electrocardiogram (ECG): A very common test for all forms of heart disease. Electrodes are placed on the chest, wrists, and ankles to record electrical signals from the heart. Unlike the echocardiogram, the ECG does not produce a structural image of heart structure.

Electrophysiological study (EPS): With this specialized test, catheters are introduced into the heart during cardiac catheterization. These catheters can both record and stimulate the electrical activity of the heart.

Ejection fraction: A measure of the power of contraction attributed to the left ventricle. It refers to the fraction of blood volume ejected with a heartbeat. Normal ejection fraction (measured by either echocardiography or MRI) is more than 50% in HCM, although the average is 70%.

Endocarditis: An infection of the heart (usually of the valves) which can occur in HCM, although very rare. Bacteria in the bloodstream can adhere to the internal surface of the heart or abnormal heart structures, particularly the mitral valve in HCM, and cause an infection.

Exercise stress testing: Exercise capacity may be tested using either a treadmill or a stationary bicycle. During an exercise test, a physician and technician monitor the patient's performance as well as symptoms, ECG, and blood pressure; sometimes the consumption of oxygen is also measured.

Gadolinium: An inert contrast agent introduced during cardiac MRI studies which accumulates in areas between heart cells and can show areas in which there is a scar.

Genes and chromosomes: Genes are the code or blueprint which build all the tissues in the body. Each individual has thousands of genes and they are all present in every cell of the body.

Genes come in pairs, one inherited from the mother and the other from the father. In each cell, the genes are grouped together by tiny, threadlike structures called chromosomes. Each person has 23 pairs of chromosomes.

HCMA: The Hypertrophic Cardiomyopathy Association is a patient support and advocacy organization. More information is available at www.4HCM.org.

Heart attack: Not appropriate terminology to describe a sudden collapse in HCM, but rather is common terminology for an acute myocardial infarction due to coronary artery disease.

Heart block: Occasionally, the normal electrical signal cannot travel into the ventricles due to a pathologic disruption in the conduction system; a slow heart rate results. This situation can be identified by an ECG and corrected with a pacemaker.

HOCM: Acronym for "hypertrophic obstructive cardiomyopathy," which is still commonly used in the United Kingdom. However, this term implies that the disease is always characterized by stenosis and outflow obstruction, which, of course, is not the case.

Holter monitor: A continuous recording of the heartbeat over 24–48 hours. Adhesive electrodes are placed on the chest, with wires that connect to a special cassette recorder which is worn on a belt. A Holter monitor detects irregularity of the heartbeat, otherwise known as arrhythmia.

Hypertrophy: Literally means an increase in the muscle mass (or weight) of the heart. In HCM, hypertrophy refers specifically to an excessive thickening of the left ventricular wall.

Hypertension: Abnormally elevated blood pressure. If not treated or controlled, can adversely affect the coronary arteries and heart, as well as the kidneys and other organs.

IHSS: Acronym for "idiopathic hypertrophic subaortic stenosis," which is an older name for HCM, used primarily in the United States in the 1960s.

Of course, this term implies that the disease is always characterized by stenosis (i.e., outflow obstruction), which is erroneous.

Implantable cardioverter defibrillator (ICD): A specialized and sophisticated device which is permanently implanted. It senses when the heart rate is excessively fast (which may represent a potentially lethal arrhythmia) and responds by either delivering a low-energy electrical shock or pacing the heart to restore the normal heart rhythm. ICDs can also serve as a pacemaker to pace the heart when the heart rate is too slow. Nevertheless, the ICD should not be confused with the conventional pacemaker. These are very different instruments with different objectives.

Mitral regurgitation: Refers to blood leaking back through the mitral valve during ejection. This occurs very commonly in HCM when there is outflow tract obstruction.

Murmur: A murmur is caused by turbulent blood flow within the heart. In HCM, the murmur is usually due to outflow obstruction and the turbulence produced by systolic anterior motion of the mitral valve or the associated mitral regurgitation. Not all murmurs, however, are of significance in patients with HCM and your doctor may regard your murmur as "innocent" and unrelated to the disease.

Mutation: A genetic defect that causes a change in the normal DNA code.

Myectomy: An operation which may be performed in severely symptomatic patients with HCM to remove a portion of the thickened muscle from the upper portion of the ventricular septum, thereby relieving the outflow tract obstruction. This procedure is usually associated with long-lasting improvement of symptoms.

Myocardial disarray: When heart tissue from patients with HCM is viewed under a microscope, the normal parallel alignment of the muscle cells (myocytes) is usually absent. Instead, characteristic of HCM, these cells (or bundles of cells) appear disorganized, or in disarray, that is, arranged at perpendicular and oblique angles to each other. There is no clinical test that can specifically detect disarray.

Myocardium: The specialized muscle which makes up the walls of the heart. It is this part of the heart which is most abnormal in HCM.

Myosin: A protein within muscle cells which is prominently involved in normal contraction. In HCM, the gene that is responsible for coding myosin is abnormal and accounts for the disease in some families.

Noninvasive: Refers to tests that generally do not invade the integrity of the body, such as echocardiography or electrocardiography. Cardiac catheterization, in which catheters are introduced through blood vessels into the heart, is an example of an invasive test.

Outflow tract: The short channel in the heart through which blood ultimately passes from the left ventricle into the aorta. It is essentially the upper portion of the left ventricle.

Outflow obstruction: Produced by the contact between mitral valve and thickened ventricular septum during the ejection phase of the heart cycle. This results in a pressure *gradient* between the upper and lower portions of the left ventricular cavity and high pressures within the left ventricular chamber. Therefore, the terms *gradient* and *obstruction* are used synonymously.

Pacemaker: When the normal electrical impulse fails to be transmitted to the ventricles, a pacemaker can be implanted to correct this problem. This involves inserting a small box containing a battery under the skin in the chest area, connected to fine wires which are inserted into a vein and to the heart, in order to deliver the necessary impulses.

Palpitation: An uncomfortable awareness of the heartbeat or rhythm. Palpitations may be due to normal heartbeats made more prominent by anxiety or exercise, or may in fact be caused by an arrhythmia. The presence of palpitations does not necessarily convey any prognostic significance in HCM, although on occasion (particularly when prolonged) they may be important signs about which you should alert your doctor.

Preimplantation genetic diagnostics (PGD): A reproductive technology used with an *in vitro* fertilization cycle. PGD can be used for diagnosis of a genetic disease in early embryos prior to implantation and pregnancy.

Septum (ventricular septum): That portion of the heart wall which divides the cavities of the right and left ventricles. In HCM, muscle thickening is usually most marked and most common in the septum. This observation has led to the descriptive term "asymmetric septal hypertrophy."

Systole: The phase of the heart cycle when blood is forcibly ejected from the ventricles – that is, blood in the left ventricle flows into the aorta and to the major arteries and organs of the body.

Systolic anterior motion of the mitral valve (SAM): In some patients with HCM, the mitral valve moves forward and touches the septum (there should normally be a considerable gap between these structures) during the ejection of blood from the heart, thereby partially blocking the flow of blood from the outflow tract into the aorta. In the vast majority of patients, SAM is the mechanism of obstruction in HCM.

Ventricles: The two main (lower) pumping chambers of the heart; the right and left ventricle pump blood to the lungs and aorta, respectively. The left ventricle is that portion of the heart most commonly and predominantly affected in HCM.

Ventricular tachycardia: A potentially serious arrhythmia in which repetitive and rapid premature beats arise within the ventricles.

Further reading

1 Maron BJ, Maron MS. Hypertrophic cardiomyopathy. Lancet 2013;381:242–255.

2 Maron BJ, Braunwald E. Evolution of hypertrophic cardiomyopathy to a contemporary treatable disease. Circulation 2012;126:1640–1644.

3 Maron BJ, Maron MS, Wigle ED, Braunwald E. The 50-year history, controversy, and clinical implications of left ventricular outflow tract obstruction in hypertrophic cardiomyopathy: from idiopathic hypertrophic subaortic stenosis to hypertrophic cardiomyopathy. J Am Coll Cardiol 2009;54:191–200.

4 Maron BJ, Maron MS, Semsarian C. Genetics of hypertrophic cardiomyopathy after 20 years: clinical perspectives. J Am Coll Cardiol 2012;60:705–715.

5 Gersh BJ, Maron BJ, Bonow RO, Dearani JA, Fifer MA, Link MS, Naidu SS, Nishimura RA, Ommen SR, Rawkowski H, Seidman CE, Towbin JA, Udelson JE, Yancy CW. 2011 ACCF/AHA guidelines for the diagnosis and treatment of hypertrophic cardiomyopathy. A report of the American College of Cardiology Foundation/American Heart Association Task Force on Practice Guidelines. Circulation 2011;124:e783–e831. J Am Coll Cardiol 2011;58:e212–e260.

6 Maron BJ, Olivotto I. Hypertrophic cardiomyopathy. In *Braunwald's Heart Disease: A Textbook of Cardiovascular Medicine*, 10th ed, Mann DK, Zipes DR, Libby P, Bonow RO (Eds). Elsevier, Philadelphia (2013).

7 Maron BJ, Spirito P, Shen W-K, Haas TS, Formisano F, Link MS, Epstein AE, Almquist AK, Daubert JP, Lawrenz T, Boriani G, Estes NAM III, Favale S, Piccininno M, Winters SL, Santini M, Betocchi S, Arribas F, Sherrid MV, Buja G, Semsarian C, Bruzzi P. Implantable cardioverter-defibrillators and prevention of sudden cardiac death in hypertrophic cardiomyopathy. JAMA 2007;298:405–412.

8 Maron BJ, Spirito P, Ackerman MJ, Casey SA, Semsarian C, Estes NAM III, Shannon KM, Ashley EA, Day SM, Anastasakis A, Bos JM, Woo A, Autore C, Pass RH, Boriani G, Garberich RF, Almquist AK, Russell MW, Boni L, Berger SN, Maron MS, Link MS. Prevention of sudden cardiac death with the implantable cardioverter-defibrillator in children and adolescents with hypertrophic cardiomyopathy. J Am Coll Cardiol 2013;61(14):1527–1535.

9 Maron BJ, Rowin EJ, Casey SA, Haas TS, Chan RHM, Udelson JE, Garberich RF, Lesser JR, Appelbaum E, Manning WJ, Maron MS. Risk stratification and outcome of

A Guide to Hypertrophic Cardiomyopathy: For Patients, Their Families, and Interested Physicians, Third Edition. Barry J. Maron and Lisa Salberg.
© 2014 John Wiley & Sons, Ltd. Published 2014 by John Wiley & Sons, Ltd.

patients with hypertrophic cardiomyopathy over 60 years of age. Circulation 2013;127:585–593.

10 Maron BJ. Contemporary insights and strategies for risk stratification and prevention of sudden death in hypertrophic cardiomyopathy. Circulation 2010;121:445–456.

11 Seidman CE, Seidman JG. Identifying sarcomere gene mutations in hypertrophic cardiomyopathy: a personal history. Circ Res 2011;108:743–750.

12 Maron BJ, Thompson PD, Ackerman MJ, Balady G, Berger S, Cohen D, Dimeff R, Douglas PS, Glover DW, Hutter AM Jr, Krauss MD, Maron MS, Mitten MJ, Roberts WO, Puffer JC. Recommendations and considerations related to preparticipation screening for cardiovascular abnormalities in competitive athletes: update 2007. A scientific statement from the American Heart Association, Nutrition, Physical Activity, and Metabolism Council. Circulation 2007;115:1643–1655.

13 Maron BJ. Hypertrophic cardiomyopathy centers. Am J Cardiol 2009;104: 1158–1159.

14 Chan RH, Maron BJ, Olivotto I, Assenza GE, Lesser JR, Haas T, Gruner C, Crean A, Rakowski H, Udelson JE, Rowin E, Tomberli B, Spirito P, Formisano F, Biagini E, Rapezzi C, De Cecco CN, Autore C, Cook EF, Hong SN, Gibson CM, Manning WJ, Appelbaum E, Maron MS. Prognostic utility of contrast-enhanced cardiovascular magnetic resonance imaging in hypertrophic cardiomyopathy: an international multicenter study (Abstract). Circulation 2012;126:A13139.

15 Harris KM, Spirito P, Maron MS, Zenovich AG, Formisano F, Lesser JR, Mackey-Bojack S, Manning WJ, Udelson JE, Maron BJ. Prevalence, clinical profile and significance of left ventricular remodeling in the end-stage phase of hypertrophic cardiomyopathy. Circulation 2006;114:216–225.

16 Maron BJ, Towbin JA, Thiene G, Antzelevitch C, Corrado D, Arnett D, Moss AJ, Seidman CE, Young JB. Contemporary definitions and classification of the cardiomyopathies. An American Heart Association Scientific Statement. Circulation 2006;113:1807–1816.

17 Maron MS, Olivotto I, Zenovich AG, Link MS, Pandian NG, Kuvin JT, Nistri S, Cecchi F, Udelson JE, Maron BJ. Hypertrophic cardiomyopathy is predominantly a disease of left ventricular outflow tract obstruction. Circulation 2006;114:2232–2239.

18 Maron BJ. The 2009 international hypertrophic cardiomyopathy summit. Am J Cardiol 2010;105:1164–1168.

19 Maron BJ. Dr. Gunnar Thor Gunnarsson and hypertrophic cardiomyopathy: what "giving back" means. Am J Cardiol 2010:105:277–278.

20 Maron BJ, Lever H. In defense of antimicrobial prophylaxis for prevention of infective endocarditis in patients with hypertrophic cardiomyopathy. J Am Coll Cardiol 2009;54:2339–2340.

21 Maron BJ. Sudden death in young athletes. N Engl Med 2003;349:1064–1075.

22 Maron BJ, Pelliccia A. The heart of trained athletes: cardiac remodeling and the risks of sports, including sudden death. Circulation 2006;114:1633–1644.

23 Maron BJ. Controversies in cardiovascular medicine. Surgical myectomy remains the primary treatment option for severely symptomatic patients with obstructive hypertrophic cardiomyopathy. Circulation 2007;116:196–206.

24 Maron BJ, Ackerman MJ, Nishimura RA, Pyeritz RE, Towbin JA, Udelson JE. Task force 4: Hypertrophic cardiomyopathy and other cardiomyopathies, mitral valve prolapse, myocarditis and Marfan syndrome. In 36th Bethesda conference. Eligibility

recommendations for competitive athletes with cardiovascular abnormalities (Maron BJ, Zipes DP). J Am Coll Cardiol 2005;45:1340–1345.

25 Maron BJ, Doerer JJ, Haas TS, Tierney DM, Mueller FO. Sudden deaths in young competitive athletes: analysis of 1866 deaths in the U.S., 1980–2006. Circulation 2009;119:1085–1092.

26 Maron BJ, Zipes DP. 36th Bethesda conference: eligibility recommendations for competitive athletes with cardiovascular abnormalities. J Am Coll Cardiol 2005;45:1312–1375.

27 Hauser RG, Maron BJ. Lessons from the failure and recall of an implantable cardioverter defibrillator. Circulation 2005;112:2040–2042.

28 Rickers C, Wilke NM, Jerosch-Herold M, Casey SA, Panse P, Panse N, Weil J, Zenovich AG, Maron BJ. Utility of cardiac magnetic resonance imaging in the diagnosis of hypertrophic cardiomyopathy. Circulation 2005;112:855–861.

29 Sherrid MV, Barac I, McKenna WJ, Elliott PM, Dickie S, Chojnowska L, Casey S, Maron BJ. Multicenter study of the efficacy and safety of disopyramide in obstructive hypertrophic cardiomyopathy. Am Coll Cardiol. 2005;45:1251–2358.

30 Maron BJ. Surgery for hypertrophic obstructive cardiomyopathy: alive and quite well. Circulation 2005;111:2016–2018.

31 Ommen SR, Maron BJ, Olivotto I, Maron MS, Cecchi F, Betocchi S, Gersh BJ, Ackerman MJ, McCully RB, Dearani JA, Schaff HV, Danielson GK, Tajik AJ, Nishimura RA. Long-term effects of surgical septal myectomy on survival in patients with obstructive hypertrophic cardiomyopathy. Am Coll Cardiol 2005;46:470–476.

32 Woo A, Williams WG, Choi R, Wigle ED, Rozenblyum E, Fedwick K, Siu S, Ralph-Edwards A, Rakowski H. Clinical and echocardiographic determinants of long-term survival after surgical myectomy in obstructive hypertrophic cardiomyopathy. Circulation 2005;111:2033–2041.

33 Nishimura RA, Holmes DR. Hypertrophic obstructive cardiomyopathy. N Engl J Med 2004;350:1320–1327.

34 Maron BJ. Hypertrophic cardiomyopathy: an important global disease (editorial). Am J Med 2004;116:63–65.

35 Maron BJ, Barry JA, Poole RS. Pilots, hypertrophic cardiomyopathy and issues of aviation and public safety. Am J Cardiol 2004;93:441–444.

36 Maron BJ, Dearani JA, Ommen SR, Maron MS, Schaff HV, Gersh BJ, Nishimura RA. The case for surgery in obstructive hypertrophic cardiomyopathy. J Am Coll Cardiol 2004;44:2044–2053.

37 Kitaoka H, Doi Y, Casey SA, Hitomi N, Furuno T, Maron BJ. Comparison of prevalence of apical hypertrophic cardiomyopathy in Japan and the United States. Am J Cardiol 2003;92:1183–1186.

38 Maron BJ. Hypertrophic cardiomyopathy: a systematic review. JAMA 2002; 287:1308–1320.

39 Olivotto I, Cecchi F, Casey SA, Dolara A, Traverse JH, Maron BJ. Impact of atrial fibrillation on the clinical course of hypertrophic cardiomyopathy. Circulation 2001;104:2517–2524.

40 Maron BJ, Gardin JM, Flack JM, Gidding SS, Kurosaki TT, Bild DE. Prevalence of hypertrophic cardiomyopathy in a general population of young adults. Echocardiographic analysis of 4111 subjects in the CARDIA study. Coronary artery risk development in (young) adults. Circulation 1995;92:785–789.

41 Spirito P, Bellone P, Harris KM, Bernabo P, Bruzzi P, Maron BJ. Magnitude of left ventricular hypertrophy and risk of sudden death in hypertrophic cardiomyopathy. N Engl J Med 2000;342:1778–1785.

42 Maron BJ, Nishimura RA, McKenna WJ, Rakowski H, Josephson ME, Kieval RS. Assessment of permanent dual-chamber pacing as a treatment for drug-refractory symptomatic patients with obstructive hypertrophic cardiomyopathy. A randomized, double-blind, crossover study (M-PATHY). Circulation 1999;99:2927–2933.

43 Maron BJ, Braunwald E. Eugene Braunwald MD and the early years of hypertrophic cardiomyopathy: a conversation with Dr. Barry J. Maron. Am J Cardiol 2012; 109:1539–1547.

44 Maron BJ, Seidman CE, Ackerman MJ, Towbin JA, Maron MS, Ommen SR, Nishimura RA, Gersh BJ. How should hypertrophic cardiomyopathy be classified?: What's in a name? Dilemmas in nomenclature characterizing hypertrophic cardio-myopathy and left ventricular hypertrophy. Circ Cardiovasc Genet 2009;2:81–85.

45 Landstrom AP, Ackerman MJ. Mutation type is not clinically useful in predicting prognosis in hypertrophic cardiomyopathy. Circulation 2010;122:2441–2449.

46 Olivotto I, Maron MS, Adabag AS, Casey SA, Vargiu D, Link MS, Udelson JE, Cecchi F, Maron BJ. Gender-related differences in the clinical presentation and outcome of hypertrophic cardiomyopathy. J Am Coll Cardiol 2005;46:480–487.

47 Ho CY. Genetics and clinical destiny: improving care in hypertrophic cardiomyopa-thy. Circulation 2010;122:2430–2440.

48 Maron BJ, Yeates L, Semsarian C. Clinical challenges of genotype positive (+)-phenotype negative (−) family members in hypertrophic cardiomyopathy. Am J Cardiol 2011;107:604–608.

49 Maron BJ, Casey SA, Haas TS, Kitner CL, Garberich RF, Lesser JR. Hypertrophic car-diomyopathy with longevity to 90 years or older. Am J Cardiol 2012;109:1341–1347.

50 Maron MS, Kalsmith BM, Udelson JE, Li W, DeNofrio D. Survival after cardiac trans-plantation in patients with hypertrophic cardiomyopathy. Circ Heart Fail 2010;3:574–579.

51 Spirito P, Autore C, Rapezzi C, Bernabò P, Badagliacca R, Maron MS, Bongioanni S, Coccolo F, Estes NA, Barillà CS, Biagini E, Quarta G, Conte MR, Bruzzi P, Maron BJ. Syncope and risk of sudden death in hypertrophic cardiomyopathy. Circulation 2009;119:1703–1710.

52 Maron BJ, Yacoub M, Dearani JA. Controversies in cardiovascular medicine. Benefits of surgery in obstructive hypertrophic cardiomyopathy: bring septal myectomy back for European patients. Eur Heart J 2011;32:1055–1058.

53 ten Cate FJ, Soliman OI, Michels M, Theuns DA, de Jong PL, Geleijnse ML, Serruys PW. Long-term outcome of alcohol septal ablation in patients with obstructive hyper-trophic cardiomyopathy: a word of caution. Circ Heart Fail 2010;3:362–369.

54 Maron MS, Maron BJ, Harrigan C, Buros J, Gibson CM, Olivotto I, Biller L, Lesser JR, Udelson JE, Manning WJ, Appelbaum E. Hypertrophic cardiomyopathy phenotype revisited after 50 years with cardiovascular magnetic resonance. J Am Coll Cardiol 2009;54:220–228.

55 Maron MS, Olivotto I, Betocchi S, Casey SA, Lesser JR, Losi MA, Cecchi F, Maron BJ. Effect of left ventricular outflow tract obstruction on clinical outcome in hyper-trophic cardiomyopathy. N Engl J Med 2003;348:295–303.

56 Maron MS, Finley JJ, Bos JM, Hauser RH, Manning WJ, Haas TS, Lesser JR, Udelson JE, Ackerman MJ, Maron BJ. Prevalence, clinical significance and natural history of left ventricular apical aneurysms in hypertrophic cardiomyopathy. Circulation 2008;118:1541–1549.

57 Maron MS. Clinical utility of cardiovascular magnetic resonance in hypertrophic cardiomyopathy. J Cardiovasc Magn Res 2012;14:13.

58 Kramer DB, Kesselheim AS, Salberg L, Brock DW, Maisel WH. Ethical and legal views regarding deactivation of cardiac implantable electrical devices in patients with hypertrophic cardiomyopathy. Am J Cardiol 2011;107:1071–1075.

59 Lampert R, Salberg L, Burg M. Emotional stress triggers symptoms in hypertrophic cardiomyopathy: a survey of the Hypertrophic Cardiomyopathy Association. Pacing Clin Electrophysiol 2010;33:1047–1053.

60 Lara AA, Salberg L. Patient advocacy: what is its role? Pacing Clin Electrophysiol 2009;32(Suppl. 2):S83–S85.

61 Brimacombe M, Walter D, Salberg L. Gender disparity in a large nonreferral-based cohort of hypertrophic cardiomyopathy patients. J Womens Health (Larchmt) 2008;17:1629–1634.

62 Maron BJ, Bonow RO, Salberg L, Roberts WC, Braunwald E. The first patient clinically diagnosed with hypertrophic cardiomyopathy. Am J Cardiol 2008; 102:1418–1420.

63 Salberg L. GINA update. J Cardiovasc Transl Res 2008;1:9–10.

64 Reineck, E, Rolston B, Bragg-Gresham J, Salberg L, Baty L, Kumar S, Wheeler MT, Ashley E, Saberi S, Day SM. Physical activity and other health behaviors in adults with hypertrophic cardiomyopathy. Am J Cardiol 2013;111(7):1034–1039.

65 Olivotto I, Maron BJ, Tomberli B, Appelbaum E, Salton C, Haas TS, Gibson CM, Nistri S, Servettini E, Chan RH, Udelson JE, Lesser JR, Cecchi F, Manning WJ, Maron MS. Impact of obesity on the phenotype and clinical course of hypertrophic cardiomyopathy. J Am Coll Cardiol 2013;62:449–457.

66 Colan SD, Lipshultz SE, Lowe AM, Sleeper LA, Messere J, Cox GF, Lurie PR, Orav EJ, Towbin JA. Epidemiology and cause specific outcome of hypertrophic cardiomyopathy in children: findings from the Pediatric Cardiomyopathy Registry. Circulation 2007;115:773–781.

67 Maron BJ, Casey SA, Haas TS, Kitner C, Garberich R. Hypertrophic cardiomyopathy with longevity to 90 years or older. Am J Cardiol 2012;109:1341–1347.

68 Maron BJ, Rowin EJ, Casey SA, Haas TS, Chan RHM, Udelson JE, Garberich RF, Lesser JR, Appelbaum E, Manning WJ, Maron MS. Risk stratification and outcome of patients with hypertrophic cardiomyopathy over 60 years of age. Circulation 2013;127:585–593.

Hypertrophic cardiomyopathy association

Membership application

Our primary objective at the HCMA is to provide support, advocacy, and education to patients, their families, the medical community, and the general public. We offer newsletters, meetings and symposiums, doctor referrals, new/improved treatment data, a fund-raising guide, and, most of all, peer support to our members. To help support the work of the HCMA we encourage you to become a member to assist us in helping those with HCM.

If you do not wish to join but feel that you can help us by making a contribution, please send your donation to the address below.

Please check the appropriate box.

☐ Annual Membership including a copy of $75.00
A Guide to Hypertrophic Cardiomyopathy:
For Patients, Families, and Interested Physicians
by Barry J. Maron, MD and Lisa Salberg

☐ Annual Renewal Membership $60.00

☐ Donation to the Hypertrophic Cardiomyopathy Association
in the amount of $.____ I would like to direct my donation to:

    ☐ General Operation
    ☐ Research Fund
    ☐ Scholarships

A Guide to Hypertrophic Cardiomyopathy: For Patients, Their Families, and Interested Physicians, Third Edition. Barry J. Maron and Lisa Salberg.
© 2014 John Wiley & Sons, Ltd. Published 2014 by John Wiley & Sons, Ltd.

Checks should be made payable to the HCMA and returned with this form to:

HCMA

322 Green Pond Road, Suite 200	Tel: 973-983-7429
PO Box 306	Fax: 973-983-7870
Hibernia, NJ 07842	Email: support@4hcm.org
Attn: Membership	www.4hcm.org

Donations and memberships may also be done online: www.4hcm.org

DR/MR/MRS/MISS (Circle as appropriate)

Last Name _____ ____   First Name _____

Address _____

City, State, Zip _____

Email_____ Phone _____

Index

A Guide to Hypertrophic Cardiomyopathy: For Patients, Their Families, and Interested Physicians,
Third Edition. Barry J. Maron and Lisa Salberg.
© 2014 John Wiley & Sons, Ltd. Published 2014 by John Wiley & Sons, Ltd.

Printed and bound by CPI Group (UK) Ltd, Croydon, CR0 4YY

09/10/2024

14571430-0004

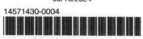